Department of Veterans Affairs
Health Services Research & Development Service | Evidence-based Synthesis Program

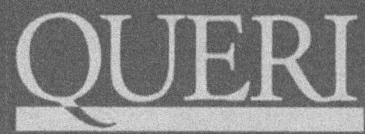

Treatment of Metastatic Non-Small Cell Lung Cancer: A Systematic Review of Comparative Effectiveness and Cost-Effectiveness

October 2012

Prepared for:
Department of Veterans Affairs
Veterans Health Administration
Quality Enhancement Research Initiative
Health Services Research & Development Service
Washington, DC 20420

Prepared by:
Evidence-based Synthesis Program (ESP) Center
West Los Angeles VA Medical Center
Los Angeles, CA
Paul G. Shekelle, M.D., Ph.D., Director

Investigators:
Principal Investigators:
Paul G. Shekelle, M.D., Ph.D.
Alicia R. Maher, M.D.

Research Associates:
Isomi M. Miake-Lye, B.A.
Jessica M. Beroes, B.S.

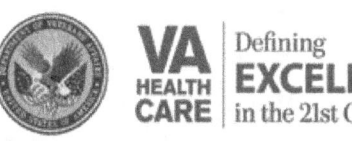

PREFACE

Quality Enhancement Research Initiative's (QUERI) Evidence-based Synthesis Program (ESP) was established to provide timely and accurate syntheses of targeted healthcare topics of particular importance to Veterans Affairs (VA) managers and policymakers, as they work to improve the health and healthcare of Veterans. The ESP disseminates these reports throughout VA.

QUERI provides funding for four ESP Centers and each Center has an active VA affiliation. The ESP Centers generate evidence syntheses on important clinical practice topics, and these reports help:
- develop clinical policies informed by evidence,
- guide the implementation of effective services to improve patient outcomes and to support VA clinical practice guidelines and performance measures, and
- set the direction for future research to address gaps in clinical knowledge.

In 2009, the ESP Coordinating Center was created to expand the capacity of QUERI Central Office and the four ESP sites by developing and maintaining program processes. In addition, the Center established a Steering Committee comprised of QUERI field-based investigators, VA Patient Care Services, Office of Quality and Performance, and Veterans Integrated Service Networks (VISN) Clinical Management Officers. The Steering Committee provides program oversight, guides strategic planning, coordinates dissemination activities, and develops collaborations with VA leadership to identify new ESP topics of importance to Veterans and the VA healthcare system.

Comments on this evidence report are welcome and can be sent to Nicole Floyd, ESP Coordinating Center Program Manager, at nicole.floyd@va.gov.

Recommended citation: Maher, AR, Miake-Lye, IM, Beroes, JM, Shekelle, PG. Treatment of Metastatic Non-Small Cell Lung Cancer: A Systematic Review of Comparative Effectiveness and Cost-Effectiveness. VA-ESP Project #05-226; 2012.

This report is based on research conducted by the Evidence-based Synthesis Program (ESP) Center located at the West Los Angeles VA Medical Center, Los Angeles, CA funded by the Department of Veterans Affairs, Veterans Health Administration, Office of Research and Development, Quality Enhancement Research Initiative. The findings and conclusions in this document are those of the author(s) who are responsible for its contents; the findings and conclusions do not necessarily represent the views of the Department of Veterans Affairs or the United States government. Therefore, no statement in this article should be construed as an official position of the Department of Veterans Affairs. No investigators have any affiliations or financial involvement (e.g., employment, consultancies, honoraria, stock ownership or options, expert testimony, grants or patents received or pending, or royalties) that conflict with material presented in the report

TABLE OF CONTENTS

EXECUTIVE SUMMARY
Background 1
Methods 1
Data Synthesis 2
Peer Review 2
Results 2
Abbreviations Table 4

INTRODUCTION 5

METHODS
Topic Development 6
Search Strategy 6
Study Selection 7
Data Abstraction 7
Quality Assessment 8
Data Synthesis 8
Rating the Body of Evidence 9
Peer Review 9

RESULTS
Literature Flow 10
Key Question #1. For patients with metastatic non-small cell lung cancer (NSCLC) what is the comparative effectiveness of the different recommended (e.g. NCCN guidelines) first line chemotherapy regimens? 11

    Key Sub-question 1.1. Does doublet chemotherapy consisting of a platinum agent plus a new agent improve outcomes compared with doublets using older agents? 13

    Key Sub-question 1.2. Does doublet chemotherapy consisting of a platinum agent plus a new agent improve outcomes compared with a new single agent alone or to a platinum agent alone? 14

    Key Sub-question 1.3. Which doublet chemotherapy regimen consisting of a platinum agent plus a new agent is most effective in improving clinical outcomes? 14

    Key Sub-question 1.4. Does doublet chemotherapy consisting of a platinum agent plus a new agent improve outcomes compared with nonplatinum combination chemotherapy including a new agent? 16

    Key Sub-question 1.5. Are new doublets containing cisplatin more effective than doublets containing carboplatin? 18

    Key Sub-question 1.6. Does triplet chemotherapy consisting of a platinum agent plus a new agent improve clinical outcomes compared with doublet chemotherapy consisting of a platinum agent plus a new agent? 18

    Key Sub-question 1.7. Does the addition of targeted therapy to doublet chemotherapy consisting of a platinum agent plus a new agent improve outcomes compared with doublet chemotherapy consisting of a platinum agent and a new agent? 19

    Key Sub-question 1.8. Is a single new agent superior to best supportive care? 23

Key Sub-question 1.9. Is a single new agent superior to single-agent or doublet therapy including older agents? 23

Key Sub-question 1.10. Which single new agent is most effective? 23

Key Sub-question 1.11. What is the optimal administration, duration, and timing of chemotherapy for advanced NSCLC? 23

Key Sub-question 1.12. Is a doublet regimen better than a single agent for the elderly population? 24

Key Sub-question 1.13. Toxicity of first-line systemic chemotherapy regimens 25

Key Question 2. For patients with metastatic NSCLC what is the comparative effectiveness of the different recommended (e.g. NCCN guidelines) second line chemotherapy regimens? 26

    Existing Systematic Reviews 26

    Clinical Trials Published Since 2006 32

    Toxicity of Second Line or Maintenance Agents 37

Key Question 3. For patients with metastatic NSCLC what is the benefit of maintenance therapy following first line chemotherapy regimens compared with no maintenance therapy? 37

Key Question 4. What is the relative cost and cost-effectiveness of the different approaches in Key Questions 1-3? 43

Key Sub-question 4.1. Which platinum-doublet is the most cost-effective therapy in squamous and in non-squamous histology types? 46

Key Sub-question 4.2. In non-squamous NSCLC, is the carboplatin-paclitaxel-bevacizumab option more cost-effective than platinum-pemetrexed? 47

Key Sub-question 4.3 Which of the three approved agents (docetaxel, pemtrexed for non-squamous histology, or erlotinib) is more cost-effective? 47

Key Sub-question 4.4. Which approach is more cost-effective: switch maintenance with pemetrexed, continuation maintenance therapy with pemetrexed or erlotinib? 49

SUMMARY AND DISCUSSION

Summary of Evidence by Key Question 51

Limitations 53

Summary 53

Recommendations for Future Research 53

REFERENCES 54

TABLES

Table F1. New Doublets vs. Older Doublets 13

Table F2. Comparison of Doublets of New Agents in Combination with Platinum Analogues 15

Table F3. New Platinum-Based Doublets vs. New Nonplatinum-Based Doublets 17

Table F4. Targeted Agents 21

Table F5. Targeted Monotherapy 22

Table F6. Summary of Grade 3 or 4 Chemotherapy Toxicity (% Patients) from Large, Selected Trials in NSCLC 25

Table S1. Second Line Systematic Reviews Published Since 2010 29

Table S2. Second Line Trials Appearing in a Systematic Review 33

Table S3. Trials Not Included in Existing Systematic Reviews 36

Table S4. Summary of Grade 3 or 4 Chemotherapy Toxicity (% Patients) from Large, Selected Trials of Maintenance or Second-line therapy 37

Table M1.	Maintenance Systematic Reviews Published Since 2010	38
Table M2.	Trials Not Included in Existing Systematic Reviews	42
Table CE1.	Cost-Effectiveness Analyses Published Since 2010	44

FIGURES

Figure 1.	A Summary of GRADE's Approach to Rating Quality of Evidence	9
Figure 2.	Literature Flow	11

APPENDIX A. SEARCH STRATEGY FOR SYSTEMATIC REVIEWS AND COST-EFFECTIVENESS ANALYSES (SEARCH #1) 71

APPENDIX B. SEARCH STRATEGY FOR TRIALS (SEARCH #2) 73

APPENDIX C. SCREENER FORMS USED FOR SYSTEMATIC REVIEWS AND COST-EFFECTIVENESS ANALYSES 75

APPENDIX D. PEER REVIEWER COMMENTS AND RESPONSES 77

EXECUTIVE SUMMARY

BACKGROUND

Lung cancer is the leading cause of cancer death in both men and women in the United States. Most patients with lung cancer are diagnosed when the cancer is already advanced (stage III or IV), and they are no longer candidates for surgical resection. Small cell lung cancer and non-small cell lung cancer (NSCLC) are treated as different diseases in terms of therapy. In the last few years, several novel agents aimed at specific molecular targets have been developed. This review was requested to evaluate the current evidence on the effectiveness and cost-effectiveness of treatments for advanced NSCLC.

The key questions were:

Key Question #1. For patients with metastatic non-small cell lung cancer (NSCLC) what is the comparative effectiveness of the different recommended (e.g. NCCN guidelines) first line chemotherapy regimens?

Key Question #2. For patients with metastatic NSCLC what is the comparative effectiveness of the different recommended (e.g. NCCN guidelines) second line chemotherapy regimens?

Key Question #3. For patients with metastatic NSCLC what is the benefit of maintenance therapy following first line chemotherapy regimens compared with no maintenance therapy?

Key Question #4. What is the relative cost and cost-effectiveness of the different approaches in Key Questions 1-3?

METHODS

We employed a two-step search strategy. The first step was to identify recently published systematic reviews; we searched PubMed and Cochrane databases for systematic reviews and cost-effectiveness analyses from 1/1/1966 through 3/16/2012, using standard search terms relating to advanced non-small cell lung cancer and cost-effectiveness analyses. The second step was to identify relevant clinical trials, which we identified by searching Medline (OVID), Embase, and Cochrane Register of Controlled Trials from 1/1/2007 through 5/8/2012, using search terms such as randomized controlled trial, carcinoma, non-small-cell, gemcitabine, etc. We limited both searches to peer-reviewed, English language literature. We also obtained a list of key publications from the technical expert panel. Additionally, systematic reviews identified in the first search were reference mined for relevant trials.

For systematic reviews and cost-effectiveness analyses to be included, they either had to present a systematic review or cost-effectiveness analysis, and had to present data on metastatic NSCLC, either for a range of stages, or more specifically for stage III, IV, or advanced NSCLC. The systematic reviews also had to assess a first line, second line, or maintenance therapy. Exclusion criteria included duplicate publications, not presenting data on NSCLC, presenting data only for stage I or II NSCLC, or not capturing treatments of interest for the systematic reviews. We did not exclude studies based solely on having assessed a drug not in current NCCN guidelines, as guidelines can change and in part do so in response to systematic reviews of evidence. To be included trials had to address first line, second line, or maintenance therapy for advanced non-small cell lung cancer.

DATA SYNTHESIS

For Key Question #1 (first-line therapy), we identified an existing systematic review which was both comprehensive and good quality, and used this article as the basis for presenting data pertinent to first-line therapy. This report was divided into sub-questions, into which we sorted the systematic reviews and trials identified by our search strategies. For Key Question #2 (second-line therapy), we created three evidence tables and narratively summarized the findings. The first evidence table presents data for the relevant systematic reviews, the second maps all relevant identified trials to the systematic reviews, and the final evidence table presents more detailed data for trials not included in the existing identified systematic reviews. For Key Question #3 (maintenance therapy), we identified a good quality, comprehensive recent review. Analogous to what was done for first-line therapy, we searched for new relevant trials in addition to the existing review. The first evidence table presents data for the relevant systematic reviews and the second presents data for relevant identified trials not included in the existing systematic reviews. For Key Question #4 (cost-effectiveness analyses), evidence table data are organized by therapy type. After obtaining input from our TEP, we focused on specific cost-effectiveness analyses of greatest interest.

PEER REVIEW

A draft version of this report was reviewed by four technical experts, as well as clinical leadership. Reviewer comments were addressed and our responses were incorporated in the final report.

RESULTS

We screened 736 titles for systematic reviews and cost-effectiveness analyses and 820 titles for trials. We screened 88 potential systematic reviews and cost-effectiveness analyses in more detail. From these, we identified 55 articles for inclusion: 24 were relevant to Key Question #1, 6 were relevant to Key Question #2, 3 were relevant to Key Question #3, and 22 were cost-effectiveness analyses relevant to Key Question #4. From the trial citations, 120 were potential includes after the title screen. Of the 60 meeting final inclusion criteria, there were 43 articles relevant to Key Question #1, 14 relevant to Key Question #2, and three relevant to Key Question #3. Peer review identified ten additions, including four trials for Key Question #1, one systematic review and two trials for Key Question #2, and one update on a trial already included for Key Question #3, as well as one new trial.

Key Question 1. First-line therapy
- **Key Sub-question 1.1.** New trials continue to support the conclusion by the CCO that any differences in survival between platinum-based doublets are modest (GRADE=high).

- **Key Sub-question 1.2.** This result continues to support the conclusions by the CCO that doublet chemotherapy including a platinum agent has a higher survival rate and a higher response rate than a single agent (GRADE=high).
- **Key Sub-question 1.3.** New trials continue to support the conclusion by Goffin and colleagues that any differences in outcomes between platinum-based agents are modest (GRADE=high).
- **Key Sub-question 1.4.** New trials continue to support the conclusion by the CCO that doublet chemotherapy including a platinum agent probably has a slight advantage over nonplatinum doublets (GRADE=moderate).
- **Key Sub-question 1.5.** One new trial does not alter the conclusion by the CCO that cisplatin combinations may have a slight advantage over carboplatin combinations in terms of survival and response rate. However, carboplatin generally has a milder toxicity than cisplatin (GRADE=moderate).
- **Key Sub-question 1.6.** New trials continue to support the review by the CCO that triplet cytotoxic therapy might have some slight advantages in terms of response rate but at an increased risk of toxicity (GRADE=high).
- **Key Sub-question 1.7.** New trials of a number of novel targeted agents have so far failed to find results equivalent to the increases in progression-free survival seen with erlotinib (mostly in patients who have never smoked) and bevacizumab (in an Asian population subgroup analysis) in the CCO review (GRADE=moderate).
- **Key Sub-question 1.7.1** Erlotinib or gefitinib monotherapy is in general superior in terms of beneficial outcomes and adverse events than cytotoxic chemotherapy in patients with EGFR mutations (GRADE=high).
- **Key Sub-question 1.12.** With the exception of studies of gefitinib and erlotinib monotherapy (in patients with EGFR mutations), doublet chemotherapy probably has a slight benefit in terms of survival compared to singlet therapy, but causes more toxicity (GRADE=moderate). Also, there now has been one trial of platinum therapy in the elderly taken to completion that found a near-doubling of the proportion of patients alive at one year in the doublet therapy group compared to monotherapy.

Summary of Key Question 2: Second-line therapy

The conclusions from the relevant systematic reviews can be summarized as:

- doublet second line cytotoxic therapy might offer slight benefits in progression-free survival and response rate, not overall survival, but at a cost of increased toxicity;
- erlotinib produces modest increases in overall survival; and
- in one phase II study, the addition of bevacizumab to second line treatment resulted in improvements in survival that were not statistically significant.

The summary of these trials not included in existing systematic reviews is:

- Considering data from first line and maintenance therapy studies in addition to second line studies, there are sufficient data to support the conclusion that histology type influences the effectiveness of potential treatments. Pemetrexed is more effective in nonsquamous NSCLC, while docetaxel is more effective in squamous NSCLC (GRADE=moderate).

- Tyrosine kinase inhibitors, when used as second-line therapy in patients unselected for EGFR mutation status, produce overall survival similar to docetaxel (GRADE=strong).
- There is insufficient data to support effectiveness of other drugs, or drugs in combinations, in second-line therapy (GRADE=moderate).
- The above second line studies are typically undertaken after evidence of disease progression, and should be distinguished from mainenance therapy, which is undertaken when a patient has at least stable disease during treatment (typically four cycles).

Summary of Key Question 3: Maintenance Therapy
- Maintenance therapy improves overall survival (GRADE=high).
- Maintenance therapy with gefitinib significantly prolonged preogression-free survival compared with placebo in patients from east Asia with advanced NSCLC who achieved disease control after first-line chemotherapy (GRADE=high).
- There is insufficient evidence to reach conclusions regarding whether a continuous or a switch strategy is superior (GRADE=very low). However, two drugs have been approved for switch therapy.
- Differences in survival in placebo-controlled trials of erlotinib or cytotoxic agents are sufficiently small that head-to-head comparisons will be required before strong conclusions can be reached about comparative effectiveness.

Summary of Key Question 4: Cost-Effectiveness Analyses

There are a large number of published cost-effectiveness analyses, but approximately two-thirds of such studies are supported by the makers of the drugs being assessed. Invariably, studies supported by the makers concluded that their drug was cost-effective. Of the cost-effectiveness analyses not supported by industry, the addition of bevacizumab to first-line therapy was found in one study to be not cost-effective, erlotinib was found in one study to be marginally cost-effective, and the differences between erlotinib and docetaxel maintenance therapy were slight in another study (GRADE=low).

ABBREVIATIONS TABLE

CI	Confidence interval
HSR&D	Health Services Research and Development Service
OR	Odds ratio
P or p	Probability
VA	Veterans Affairs
VAMC	VA Medical Center
NSCLC	Non-small cell lung cancer
ECOG	Eastern Cooperative Oncology Group
EGFR	Epidermal growth factor receptor
ASCO	American Society of Clinical Oncology
TKI	Tyrosine Kinase Inhibitors

EVIDENCE REPORT

INTRODUCTION

Lung cancer is the leading cause of cancer death in both men and women in the United States, and male Veterans seeking care at VA hospitals have a much higher age-specific incidence of lung cancer than males in the general population.[1] The personal and economic significance of lung cancer has led to a vast research endeavor to try and identify new and more effective treatments. Most patients with lung cancer are diagnosed when the cancer is already advanced (stage IIIB or IV), and they are no longer candidates for surgical resection. Small cell lung cancer and non-small cell lung cancer (NSCLC) are different diseases in terms of treatment. Until recently, all therapies for advanced NSCLC were based on their cytotoxic properties. In the last few years, several novel agents aimed at specific molecular targets have been developed. This review was requested to evaluate the current evidence on the effectiveness and cost-effectiveness of treatments for advanced lung cancer.

METHODS

TOPIC DEVELOPMENT

This project was nominated by Michael J Kelley, MD, National Program Director for Oncology/MSS/PCS and Chief, Hematology/Oncology Durham VAMC, with input from a technical expert panel (TEP), including Oncology Field Advisory Committee Membership, Dr. Jennifer Malin -- Staff Physician, Oncology, West LA VA, and Dr. Apar Ganti -- Staff Physician, Oncology, Omaha VA.

The final key questions are:

Key Question #1. For patients with metastatic non-small cell lung cancer (NSCLC) what is the comparative effectiveness of the different recommended (e.g. NCCN guidelines) first line chemotherapy regimens?

Key Question #2. For patients with metastatic NSCLC what is the comparative effectiveness of the different recommended (e.g. NCCN guidelines) second line chemotherapy regimens?

Key Question #3. For patients with metastatic NSCLC what is the benefit of maintenance therapy following first line chemotherapy regimens compared with no maintenance therapy?

Key Question #4. What is the relative cost and cost-effectiveness of the different approaches in Key Questions 1-3?

SEARCH STRATEGY

Preliminary searches done by the ESP coordinating center established that there is a very large literature on this topic, including numerous systematic reviews. With this knowledge, we employed a two-step search strategy. The first step was to identify recently published systematic reviews, and then the second step was to identify relevant clinical trials published subsequent to those reviews. We did not search conference abstracts specifically, although those that were identified in databases or through peer review were eligible for inclusion.

Search #1 Systematic Reviews and Cost-Effectiveness Analyses

We searched PubMed and Cochrane databases for systematic reviews and cost-effectiveness analyses from 1/1/1966 through 3/16/2012, using standard search terms such as lung neoplasms, lung cancer, non-small-cell, non-small cell, non small cell, metastatic, metastasic, advanced, cost-effective, cost-benefit, cost analysis, and economic. We limited the search to peer-reviewed articles involving human subjects and published in the English language (Appendix A).

Search #2 New Clinical Trials

Our second search identified trials by searching Medline (OVID), Embase, and Cochrane Register of Controlled Trials from 1/1/2007 through 5/8/2012, using search terms such as randomized controlled trial, carcinoma, non-small-cell, gemcitabine, etc. We limited the search to English language (Appendix B).

Additional Strategies

We also obtained a list of key publications from the technical expert panel. Additionally, systematic reviews identified in the first search were reference mined for relevant trials.

STUDY SELECTION

For the systematic reviews and cost-effectiveness analyses, titles obtained from the first search were reviewed in descending chronological order, starting with reviews published in 2012 and continuing backward. Given that the lag between end date of a search and publication is typically one year or more, we stopped this search at 2010, in order to capture the more recent reviews. Full-text articles of potentially relevant titles were retrieved, and each article was reviewed using the appropriate screener form (either systematic review or cost-effectiveness) in Appendix C. To be included, articles either had to present a systematic review or cost-effectiveness analysis, and had to present data on metastatic NSCLC, either for a range of stages, or more specifically for stage IIIB, IV, or advanced NSCLC. The systematic reviews also had to assess a first line, second line, or maintenance therapy. Exclusion criteria included duplicate publications, not presenting data on NSCLC, presenting data only for stage I or II NSCLC, or not capturing treatments of interest for the systematic reviews.

After having reviewed the existing systematic reviews, we determined that the best available existing review used a search ending in December 2007. We therefore conducted a second search, starting in January 2007, for all relevant clinical trials. For trials identified by this second search, titles were screened for relevance. Abstracts for included titles were then sorted by type of therapy: first line, second line, or maintenance. This corresponded with the first three key questions. The articles that did not address at least one of these types of therapy were excluded. Full-text articles were then retrieved for these trials.

Some literature prior to 2007 was included in the review because it came from our TEP or peer reviewers.

DATA ABSTRACTION

We abstracted the following data for each included systematic review and cost-effectiveness analysis: Inclusion and exclusion criteria discussed above, type of therapy assessed, treatment captured/assessed, outcomes reported/used, and conclusions per abstract. For systematic reviews, we also abstracted the search end date, databases searched, and number of studies included. For cost-effectiveness analyses, we also abstracted whether the data were from a single study or multiple studies and what perspective the analysis was from (US payer, non-US payer, societal, or other).

For trials, the data abstracted depended on the Key Question, or sub-question, the article addressed. Potential types of data include: treatment/drug being assessed or compared, overall survival, response rate, sample size, study/setting, and conclusions per abstract.

QUALITY ASSESSMENT

All studies included as evidence for key questions 1-3 are randomized trials or systematic reviews of randomized trials. For practical reasons, these cannot (in general) be blinded, as the dosing regimens are different for the various agents being compared (the exception being the some of the newer targeted therapies that can be taken orally). Using conventional metrics of quality assessment (randomization, blinding, withdrawals and dropouts) will not discriminate between studies except on the follow up rate, which has been recorded where applicable in the evidence tables. Where reported, the follow up rate is usually above 80 percent. Consequently, almost all studies in key questions 1-3 are considered approximately equivalent in terms of their risk of bias, and no subgroup analysis are performed that use risk of bias as a stratifying factor.

DATA SYNTHESIS

For Key Question #1 (first-line therapy), we identified an existing systematic review from the Cancer Care Ontario Program in Evidence-Based Care (CCO) by Goffin and colleagues which was both comprehensive and good quality, and used this article as the basis for presenting data pertinent to first-line therapy.[2] This report was divided into sub-questions, into which we sorted the systematic reviews and trials identified by our search strategies #1 and #2, detailed above. When the CCO had created evidence tables for a sub-question and our search identified new information relevant to that particular sub-question, these tables were reproduced and the new trials were added. Data were then narratively summarized for all sub-questions of interest.

For Key Question #2 (second-line therapy), we created three evidence tables. The first evidence table presents data for the relevant systematic reviews, including search end date, treatments being compared, included articles, outcomes reported, and conclusions per abstract. The second evidence table presents an abbreviated citation and whether or not the article was included in any of the systematic reviews for all articles identified by the second search and the TEP. The final evidence table presents data for trials not included in the existing identified systematic reviews, including number of patients randomized, agents being compared and patients in each of these treatment groups, median survival, one year survival, and overall response. We then narratively summarized evidence within each identified group of similar trials.

For Key Question #3 (maintenance therapy), we identified a good quality, comprehensive recent review by Zhang and colleagues.[3] Analogous to what was done for first-line therapy, we searched for new relevant trials in addition to the existing review. The first evidence table presents data for the relevant systematic reviews, including search end date, treatments being compared, total trials and number of patients included, included articles, outcomes reported, and conclusions per abstract. The second evidence table presents data for trials identified by the second search and TEP that were not included in the existing systematic reviews. Data presented includes study or setting, type of therapy the maintenance is following, treatments being compared, outcomes reported, and results and conclusions per abstract.

For Key Question #4 (cost-effectiveness analyses), data are organized by therapy type (first-line therapy, second-line therapy, maintenance therapy, and other therapy). For each article, treatments assessed, data origin, analysis perspective, outcomes used, and conclusions per abstract are presented. After obtaining input from our TEP, we focused on specific cost-effectiveness analyses of greatest interest.

RATING THE BODY OF EVIDENCE

We assessed the overall quality of evidence for outcomes using a method developed by the GRADE Working Group, which classified the grade of evidence across outcomes according to the following criteria:

- High = Further research is very unlikely to change our confidence on the estimate of effect.
- Moderate = Further research is likely to have an important impact on our confidence in the estimate of effect and may change the estimate.
- Low = Further research is very likely to have an important impact on our confidence in the estimate of effect and is likely to change the estimate.
- Very Low = Any estimate of effect is very uncertain.

Figure 1. A summary of GRADE's approach to rating quality of evidence[4]

Study design	Initial quality of a body of evidence	Lower if	Higher if	Quality of a body of evidence
Randomized trials	High	Risk of Bias -1 Serious -2 Very serious Inconsistency -1 Serious -2 Very serious Indirectness -1 Serious -2 Very serious Imprecision -1 Serious -2 Very serious Publication Bias -1 Likely -2 Very likely	Large Effect +1 Large +2 Very large Dose response +1 Evidence of a gradient All plausible residual confounding +1 Would reduce a demonstrated effect +1 Would suggest a spurious effect if no effect was observed	High (four plus: ⊕⊕⊕⊕)
Observational studies	Low			Moderate (three plus: ⊕⊕⊕O)
				Low (two plus: ⊕⊕OO)
				Very low (one plus: ⊕OOO)

PEER REVIEW

A draft version of this report was reviewed by four technical experts as well as clinical leadership. Their comments and our responses are presented in Appendix D.

RESULTS

LITERATURE FLOW

From the search for systematic reviews and cost-effectiveness analyses, we received 736 titles. We narrowed the scope to systematic reviews published after 2010 during the title screen, and identified 88 potential citations for inclusion. Full articles were retrieved and screened for 55 articles. Of these, 22 were cost-effectiveness analyses relevant to Key Question #4. The remaining 33 included articles were systematic reviews of first line, second line, or maintenance therapies for advanced, stage III, or stage IV NSCLC. These were then distributed among the relevant Key Questions: 22 were relevant to Key Quest #1, 6 were relevant to Key Question #2, and 3 were relevant to Key Question #3. One additional systematic review was identified by our peer reviewers relevant to Key Question #3.

From the search for trials, we received 820 titles, and after a title screen, there were 158 citations identified for potential inclusion. From these citations, 120 articles were identified for full article screening. Of the 60 meeting the final inclusion criteria, there were 43 articles relevant to Key Question #1, 14 relevant to Key Question #2, and three relevant to Key Question #3. An additional seven trials, plus one update on a trial already included in the review, were identified by our peer reviewers and distributed as follows: four were relevant to Key Question #1, two were relevant to Key Question #2, and one trial plus the update were relevant to Key Question #3.

Figure 2 details the review process and the number of references related to each of the key questions.

Figure 2. Literature Flow

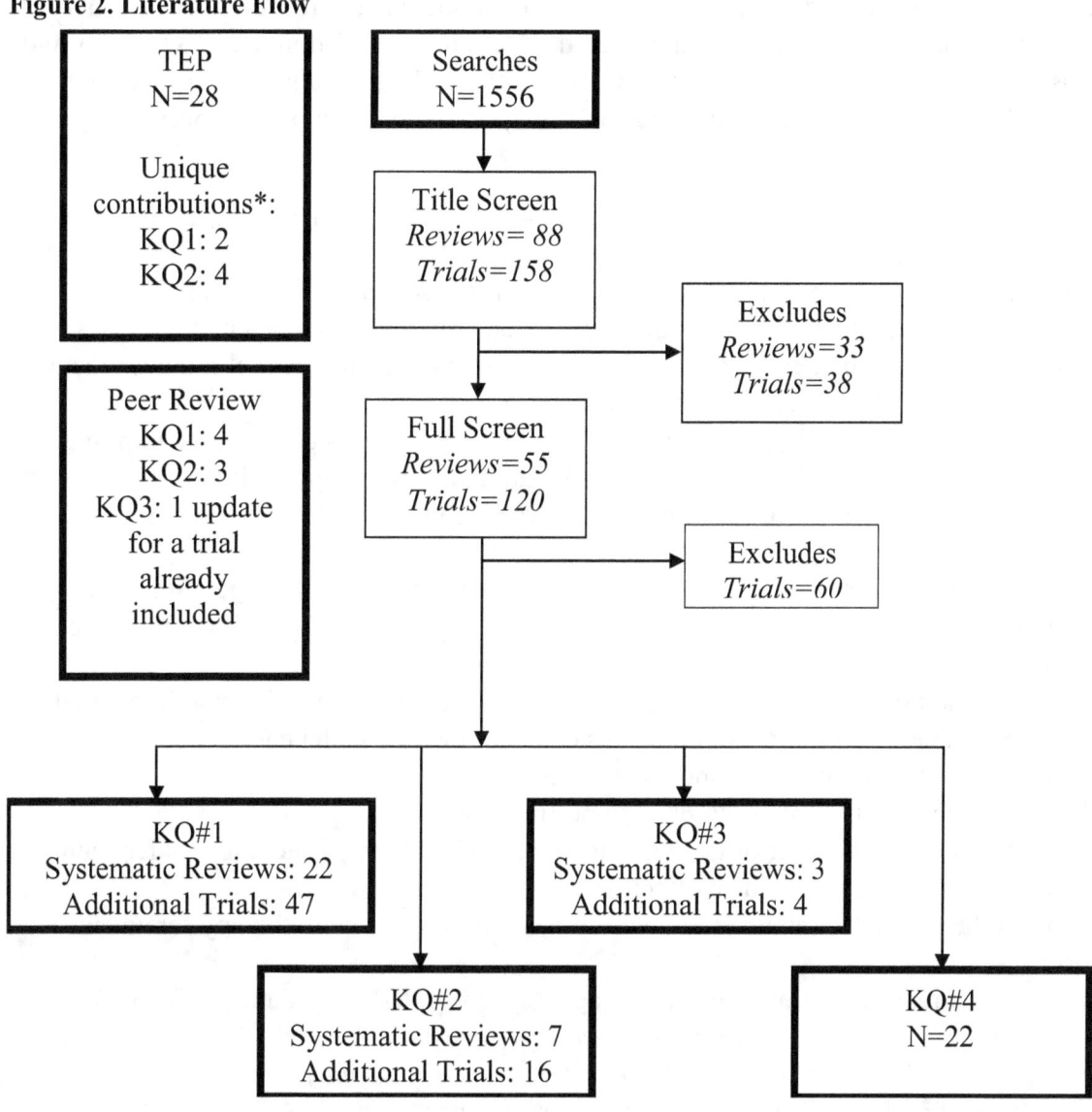

*Most TEP recommendations were already included in either a systematic review or the newly identified trials in from our search. Only the six noted above were not included from another source.

KEY QUESTION #1. For patients with metastatic non-small cell lung cancer (NSCLC) what is the comparative effectiveness of the different recommended (e.g. NCCN guidelines) first line chemotherapy regimens?

We identified 22 systematic reviews or meta-analyses published since 2010 that addressed NSCLC first-line therapy. [2, 5-25] Most of these reviews were narrowly targeted at specific questions. The most comprehensive of these reviews was published by the Cancer Care Ontario Program in Evidence-Based Care (CCO) in 2010 by Goffin and colleagues.[2] This review scored a "yes" on 9 out of 11 of the AMSTAR criteria,[26] searched multiple databases through 2007, and included 10 systematic reviews and 46 randomized trials. The CCO first searched for relevant systematic reviews, and then added new trials that were not included in those reviews. In our review we follow the same format: we summarize the literature included in the CCO review and then discuss additional trials, systematic reviews, and meta-analyses not included in this main review. The CCO review had 13 key questions, which we incorporate into this report as key sub-questions:

- Does doublet chemotherapy consisting of a platinum agent plus a new agent improve outcomes compared with doublets using older agents?
- Does doublet chemotherapy consisting of a platinum agent plus a new agent improve outcomes compared with a new single agent alone or to a platinum agent alone?
- Which doublet chemotherapy regimen consisting of a platinum agent plus a new agent is most effective in improving clinical outcomes?
- Does doublet chemotherapy consisting of a platinum agent plus a new agent improve outcomes compared with nonplatinum combination chemotherapy including a new agent?
- Are new doublets containing cisplatin more effective than doublets containing carboplatin?
- Does triplet chemotherapy consisting of a platinum agent plus a new agent improve clinical outcomes compared with doublet chemotherapy consisting of a platinum agent plus a new agent?
- Does the addition of targeted therapy to doublet chemotherapy consisting of a platinum agent plus a new agent improve outcomes compared with doublet chemotherapy consisting of a platinum agent and a new agent?
- Is a single new agent superior to best supportive case?
- Is a single new agent superior to single-agent or doublet therapy including older agents?
- Which single new agent is most effective?
- What is the optimal administration, duration, and timing of chemotherapy for advanced nsclc?
- Is a doublet regimen better than a single agent for the elderly population? *This was modified by our tep from the original question in the cco review: which single or doublet regimen including a new agent is superior for the elderly population?*
- Toxicity of first-line systemic chemotherapy regimens

The overall conclusion of the review by the CCO was that "data continue to support the use of a platinum agent plus a new agent as the reference standard."[2] They also concluded that the combination of a platinum agent and a new agent had "a slight advantage over pairs of new agents, although at the cost of greater toxicity." Cisplatin combinations were judged to have a "slight" advantage over carboplatin combinations, although carboplatin combinations had a more favorable toxicity profile. Finally, the CCO concluded that "as differences between regimens are small, toxicities and patient preference should help guide treatment choice." Data on the new targeted therapies were just emerging at the time of the CCO review. A subsequent addendum limited to pemetrexed concluded that the data "are sufficiently compelling to recommend that pemetrexed should not be used in the treatment of squamous cell carcinomas for first line treatment."

Key Sub-question 1.1. Does doublet chemotherapy consisting of a platinum agent plus a new agent improve outcomes compared with doublets using older agents?

The CCO review included one meta-analysis by Baggstrom and colleagues,[27] which itself consisted of six RCTs, and five additional RCTs.[28-32] The meta-analysis of six trials of doublet regimens found results favoring chemotherapy regimens containing platinum and a new agent, with a 1-year survival rate risk difference of 6% (95% CI: 2-10%).[27] The five additional trials comparing old to new doublet therapies, only one found superior survival with a newer agent, that being docetaxel plus cisplatin over vindesine plus cisplatin.[29]

New Literature Since 2007 Relevant to this Sub-question

Our update search identified seven new RCTs relevant to this sub-question.[33-39] Details of these studies, plus those from the CCO review, are in Table F1. Among these seven new studies, none reported significant benefit in outcomes when comparing the newer, to older, doublets. One study actually found worse outcomes with the newer agent, pemetrexed, versus the older agent, etoposide.[36] Overall survival was 8.1 months with pemetrexed, versus 10.6 months with etoposide (HR=1.56, 95% CI: 1.27-1.92; log-rank P<.01) and the objective response rate was 31% vs. 52% (P<.001).

Table F1. New Doublets vs. Older Doublets (adapted from Goffin)

Trial		Comparison		Survival (95% CI), p Value		Overall Response (95% CI), p Value
Reference	$N_{rand}/N_{eval}{}^a$	Agents	$N_{rand}/N_{eval}{}^a$	Median (mo)	1-yr %	
Belani et al.[28]	369	PCb	190	7.7 (p = 0.086)	32	23 (NR), p = 0.061
		EtC	179	9.0	37	15
Ichinose et al.[29]	311/302	DC	NR/151	11.4 (NR)	24 (NR) [2 yr]p=0.01	37 (NR), p = 0.004
		VdC	NR/151	9.6 (NR)	12 (NR)	21 (NR)
Kim et al.[30b]	75/62	GC	39/33	18.7 (NR) p = 0.29	NR	63.6 (NR), p = 0.001
		EtC	36/29	15 (NR)	NR	20.7 (NR)
Park et al.[31]	78/67	DC	40/34	NR	NR	NR
		EtC	38/33	NR	NR	NR
Takiguchi[32]	210	IrC	104	10	43	29 (28/98)
		VdC	106	11.1	48	22 (22/101)
Schmittel[33]	216	IrCb	106	10.0 (8.4-11.6)	37.1 (26.1-48.1)	54
		EtCb	110	p=0.06	p=0.36)	52
				9.0 (7.6-10.4)	30.3(20.5-40.1)	
Zatloukal[34]	407/405	IrC	202	10.2(9.0-11.7)	41.9	39.1
		EtC	203	p=0.06	38.9	46.6
				9.7(8.9-11.1)		
Yamamoto[35] (+TRT)	456/440	IrCb	152/147	19.8,p=.876	NR	56.5
		PCb	151/147	22.0	NR	63.0
		MVPVdC	153/146	20.5,p=.392	NR	66.4
Hermes[39] (+brain radiation)	209	IrCb	105	8.5	34	NR
		EtCb	104	7.1	24	NR
Dimitroulis[38]	108	PC	53	12 (11.0-13.0)	NR	71.7 (38/53) (44.99-76.07),
		EtC	55	,p=0.354	NR	p=0.815
				13(11.7-12.85)		70.9 (39/55) (42.19-73.59)
Lee[37]	241	GCb	121	8.0 (1.84-2.56)	30.6	63.3
		EtC	120	8.1	31.0	62.7
Socinski[36]	908	PemCb	453	8.1 (1.27-1.92),	26(20-32)	31
		EtCb	455	p<.01	40(33-48)	52
				10.6		

*New entries are shaded.
^{a} N_{eval} only reported when analysis was not intention-to-treat
^{b} "Preliminary results" noted. Not clear whether referring to preliminary report, or interim analysis. No other indication this is an interim analysis.
C, cisplatin; Cb, carboplatin; CI, confidence interval; D, docetaxel; Et, etoposide; G, gemcitabine; Ir, Irinotecan; N_{eval}, number of patients evaluable; N_{rand}, number of patients randomized; NR, not reported; P, paclitaxel; Vd, vindesine; MVP, mitomycin; Pem, pemetrexed

Summary of Key Sub-question 1.1

New trials continue to support the conclusion by the CCO that any differences in survival between platinum-based doublets are modest (GRADE=High).

Key Sub-question 1.2. Does doublet chemotherapy consisting of a platinum agent plus a new agent improve outcomes compared with a new single agent alone or to a platinum agent alone?

The review by the CCO included a meta-analysis by Hotta, which itself included eight trials of 2,374 patients.[40] In these trials, a doublet of platinum plus a new agent versus a new agent alone found an improvement in survival for platinum-based doublets (HR=0.87; 95% CI: 0.80-0.94; p<0.001) and a higher response rate (OR=2.32, 95% CI: 1.68-3.20) compared with new single agent therapy.

New Literature Since 2007 Relevant to this Sub-question

We identified one new published trial relevant to this Key Sub-question. Reynolds and colleagues randomized 170 patients with performance status of two to either gemcitabine or gemcitabine plus carboplatin.[41] The median survival was 6.7 (4.9-10.0) months in the gemcitabine plus carboplatin group and 5.1 (3.9-6.3) months for gemcitabine. This difference was not statistically significant (p=0.14). Overall survival at one year was 31.3 percent in the doublet therapy group and 21.2 percent in the gemcitabine alone therapy group (statistical testing not performed). There was a statistically significant higher rate of confirmed response in the gemcitabine plus carboplatin (21.1%) group compared to gemcitabine alone (6.3%, p=.01). In addition, patients' tumors were evaluated for RRM1 and ERCC1 protein levels and found that these were significantly and inversely correlated with disease response.

During peer review, we were directed to a recently presented abstract of a second relevant study[42]. Patients with advanced NSCLC and a performance status of 2 were randomized to receive pemetrexed or carboplatin plus pemetrexed. During the trial, eligibility was later restriced to only patients with nonsquamous histology. Overall survival among 205 patients studied was 9.1 months versus 5.6 months, favoring doublet therapy (p=0.001). We await full publication of these results, which provide additional support favoring doublet therapy, even in patients with a poor performance status.

Summary of Key Sub-question 1.2

This result continues to support the conclusions by the CCO that doublet chemotherapy including a platinum agent has a higher survival rate and a higher response rate than a single agent (GRADE=High).

Key Sub-question 1.3. Which doublet chemotherapy regimen consisting of a platinum agent plus a new agent is most effective in improving clinical outcomes?

The review by the CCO identified two meta-analyses[43, 44] and nine studies,[32, 45-52] three of which were included in one of the two meta-analyses.[45, 46, 50] The first meta-analysis, by Le Chevalier et al, examined the efficacy of gemcitabine plus platinum combinations versus any other platinum-based regimen.[43] Out of six trials, there was a trend toward superior survival with gemcitabine-based regimens and improved progression-free survival (HR= 0.89; 95% CI: 0.82-0.96). The second meta-analysis, by Douillard et al., compared seven trials of docetaxel-containing regimens with vinca-alkaloid regimens.[44] Docetaxel led to greater overall survival (HR=0.89; 95% CI: 0.82-0.96; P=0.004). In the nine additional studies, median survival ranged from 6.4-14.0 months, without consistent differences between arms.

New Literature Since 2007 Relevant to this Sub-question

Our search identified nine additional studies[53-61] and two subsequent meta-analyses[62, 63] relevant to this Key Sub-question. These new results did not alter the conclusions reached by the CCO. The combinations studied included gemcitabine, paclitaxel, paclitaxel poliglumex (CT-2013 PPX), S-1, pemetrexed, vinorelbine, and docetaxel. Details of these studies, as well as the studies contained in the CCO review, are in Table F2. No particular combination was shown to be significantly superior in outcomes. Median survival ranged from 7.0 to 15.2 months. Of note, the study comparing paclitaxel plus carboplatin vs. gemcitabine plus oxaliptin had to be terminated after adverse events exceeded the safety threshold set by the data safety and monitoring board.[60]

We also identified one clinical trial comparing doublet chemotherapy regimens, but neither included a platinum agent. This study compared paclitaxel and gemcitabine to paclitaxel and vinorelbine in 39+ patients with stage IIIB or IV NSCLC. There was no difference in median overall survival (11.1 months vs. 8.6 months, p=0.14); the group treated with vinorelbine had more grade 3/4 toxicities.[25]

Table F2. Comparison of Doublets of New Agents in Combination with Platinum Analogues (adapted from Goffin)

Trial		Comparison		Survival (95% CI), *p* Value		Overall Response (95% CI), *p* Value
Reference	N_{rand}/N_{eval}[a]	Agents	N_{rand}/N_{eval}[a]	Median (mo)	1-yr %	
Fossella et al.[50]	1218/—	DC	104	11.3 (10.1–12.4) p = 0.044	46 (42–51)[c]	vs. VC, 31.6 (NR) p = 0.029
		DCb	406		38 (33–43)	
		VC	404	9.4 (8.7–10.6)	40–41 (35–46)	vs. VC, 23.9 (NR) p = 0.870
				9.9–10.1 (9.0–11.3)[b]		24.5 (NR)
Gebbia et al.[49]	400/NR	GC	138/NR	8.2 (NR) p = 0.187	20 (NR) p = 0.4	33 (26–42) p = 0.032
		VC	140/NR	9.0 (NR)	24 (NR)	44 (36–53) p = 0.007[d]
		GI ->VC	62/NR	NR	NR	19 (10–31)[d]
		VC->GI	60/NR	NR	NR	32 (20–45)[d]
Helbekkmo et al.[52]	432	VCb	218	7.3 (NR) p = 0.89	28	NR
		GCb	214	6.4 (NR)	30	NR
Martoni et al.[48]	272/—	VC	137	11 (9–13) p = 0.759	39.7 (NR)	32.1 (24.5–40.5) p = 0.32
		GC	135	11 (9–13)	44.4 (NR)	26.7 (19.5–35.1)
Ohe et al.[51]	602/—	IrC	151	13.9 (NR) p = ns	59.2 (NR)[e]	31 (NR)
		PCb	150	12.3 (NR)	51.0 (NR)	32.4 (NR) p = 0.80
		GC	151	14.0 (NR)	59.6 (NR)	30.1 (NR) vs. IrC, p = 0.87
		VC	150	11.4 (NR)	48.3 (NR)	33.1 (NR) vs. IrC, p = 0.71
Rubio and Sahagun[47]	60	DCb	29	10.2 (NR) p = ns	NR	46.4 (NR)
		VCb	31	10.7 (NR)	NR	45.2 (NR)
Scagliotti et al.[46]	612/—	VC	203	9.5 (8.3–11.0)	37 (NR) p = 0.48[f]	30 (24–36) p = 0.98
		GC	205	9.8 (8.6–11.2)	37 (NR)	30 (24–37)
		PCb	204	10.0 (9.0–12.5)	43 (NR)vs.VC, p = 0.1[g]	32 (25–38) vs. VC, p = 0.75

Trial		Comparison		Survival (95% CI), *p* Value		Overall Response (95% CI), *p* Value
Reference	N_{rand}/N_{eval}[a]	Agents	N_{rand}/N_{eval}[a]	Median (mo)	1-yr %	
Schiller et al.[45]	1207/1155	PC	303/288	7.8 (7.0–8.9) p = ns	31 (26–36)	21 (NR) p = ns
		GC	301/288	8.1 (7.2–9.4)	36 (31–42)	22 (NR)
		DC	304/289	7.4 (6.6–8.8)	31 (26–36)	17 (NR)
		PCb	299/290	8.1 (7.0–9.5)	34 (29–40)	17 (NR)
Takiguchi et al.[32]	210	IrC	104	10	43	29 (28/98)
		VdC	106	11.1	48	22 (22/101)
Treat, 2010[59]	1135	GCb	379	7.9, p=0.693	33.9	25.3
		GP	377	8.5	36.2	32.1
		PCb	379	8.7	35.6	29.8
Weissman[60]	383	PCb		Study terminated after 383 patients randomized- adverse events exceeded safety threshold		
		GOx				
Kelly, 2001[64]	408	VC	202	8.1(6.7-9.6)	36	28
		PCb	206	8.6(7.2-10.7)	38	25
Okamoto[55]	564	PCb	281	13.3 (11.7-15.1)	55.5	29.0, p=.019
		S-1Cb	282	15.2 (12.4-17.1)	57.3	20.4
Rodrigues-Pereira[56]	260	PemCb	128	14.9 (12.2-10-19.0)	NR	34.0
		DCb	132	14.7 (10.8-19.8)		22.9
Scaggliotti[57]	1725	PemC	862	10.3 (0.84-1.05)	43.5	30.6
		GC	863	10.3	41.9	28.2
Chang[53]	83/73	GC	34	12.9	55.9	38 (13/34)(21-55) p=0.622
		VC	39	9.0	33.3	31 (12/31)(16-460)
Tan[58]	390/ 381	VC	190	9.9 (8.41-11.6)	39.4	31.2 (24-39)
		DC	191	9.8 (8.80-11.5)	40.9	29.6 (22.8-37)
Gronberg[54]	446	PemCb	225	7.3, p=.63	34	NR
		GCb	221	7.0	31	NR
Langer[61]	400	PxCb	199	7.8	31 (24-37)	20(15-27)
		PCb	201	7.9	31 (25-38)	37(30-44)

*New entries are shaded.

[a] N_{eval} only reported when analysis was not intention-to-treat.
[b] Survival estimates were adjusted for prognostic factors, and minor differences in the distribution of those factors produced slightly different values.
[c] The hazard ratios and 95% CI of overall survival for DC and DCb vs. VC were 97.2 (0.989 –1.416) and 97.2 (0.877–1.253), respectively.
[d] Data are from an interim analysis of 243 patients. At interim, VC response was statistically superior to GI–_VC, p _ 0.007, all other interim comparisons not significant at a 95% confidence level.
[e] This was a noninferiority trial. The difference in 1-yr survival between arms was as follows: IrC vs. PCb -8.2% (-19.6 -3.3%), PCb vs. GC 0.4% (-10.9 -11.7%), GC vs. VC -10.9% (-22.3 -0.5%). Conclusions of this trial are faulty. They report they cannot reject the null hypothesis of noninferiority, but still say agents are similar. The values reported here are the difference in 1-yr survival between agents and the IrC arm.
[f] Hazard ratio of survival was 0.87 (0.69 –1.09).
[g] Hazard ratio of survival for VC vs. PCb was 0.84 (0.67–1.05).
C, cisplatin; D, docetaxel; Cb, carboplatin; CI, confidence interval; G, gemcitabine; I, ifosfamide; Ir, irinotecan; N_{eval}, number of patients evaluable; N_{rand}, number of patients randomized; NR, not reported; ns, not significant; P, paclitaxel; V, vinorelbine; Vd, Vinblastine; Ox, oxaliptin; Px, Paclitaxel poliglumex (CT-2103 PPX)

Summary of Key Sub-question 1.3

New trials continue to support the conclusion by the CCO that any differences in outcomes between doublet therapies with platinum-based agents are modest (GRADE=High).

Key Sub-question 1.4. Does doublet chemotherapy consisting of a platinum agent plus a new agent improve outcomes compared with nonplatinum combination chemotherapy including a new agent?

The review by the CCO identified two meta-analyses and four additional relevant RCTs.[65-70] The first meta-analysis, by Pujol et al., analyzed 11 RCTs comparing platinum-based new doublets or a combination of new nonplatinum agents, in 4602 patients.[67] There was a 2.9% absolute reduction in the risk of death at 1-year with the platinum-based regimens (OR=0.88; 95% CI: 0.78-0.99, P=0.044). The other meta-analysis, by D'Addario et al, examined 14 trials and found no survival benefit with platinum-based agents over nonplatinum chemotherapy regimens (OR, 1.11; 95% CI: 0.096-1.28; P=0.17).[65] In the four additional studies, median survival ranged from 7.6 to 13.8 months.[66, 68-70] One of these studies, Tan et al, found improvement in the median survival in those patients receiving gemcitabine-vinorelbine (11.5 months) compared to those receiving vinorelbine-carboplatin (8.6 months, P=0.01).[69]

New Literature Since 2007 Relevant to this Sub-question

The additional three trials we identified did not find a significant difference between agents and did not alter the conclusions reached by the CCO.[59, 71, 72] Details of these three and the four RCTs identified by the CCO are presented in Table F3. In one of these trials, platinum-based regimens of gemcitabine or paclitaxel with carboplatin led to a median survival of 7.9 (7.1-9.2, P=0.693) and 8.7 (7.7-9.9) months, compared to gemcitabine with paclitaxel which led to 8.5 (7.6-10.0) months.[59] In another trial, the combination of gemcitabine with paclitaxel led to a median survival of 9.97 (8.74- 12.0) months compared to 10.49 months with gemcitabine and carboplatin (9.04-11.94).[72] Though the final study appeared to favor gemcitabine and epirubicin with a median survival of 21.5 months versus 13.2 months for gemcitabine-cisplatin, the confidence intervals were wide (9.4-33.6 and 10.4-16.0) and the number of patients small (80 and 85).[71]

Table F3. New Platinum-Based Doublets vs. New Nonplatinum-Based Doublets (adapted from Goffin)

Study Reference	$N_{rand}/N_{eval}{}^a$	Comparison Agents	$N_{rand}/N_{eval}{}^a$	Survival (95% CI), p Value Median (mo)	1-yr %	Overall Response (95% CI), p Value
Kawahara et al.[66]	401/393	VG->D	NR	13.1 (NR) p = 0.28	55.6 (NR)	23 (NR) p = 0.008
		PCb	NR	13.8 (NR)	55.6 (NR)	36 (NR)
Rigas et al.[68]	928	DCb	466	8.1	35	NR
		GD	463	8.3	34	NR
Tan et al.[69]	316/—	VCb	159	8.6 (NR) p = 0.01	34.4 (NR)	20.8 (NR) p = 0.15
		VG	157	11.5 (NR)	48.9 (NR)	28.0 (NR)
Treat[70]	929/788	GCb	309/265	7.6 (6.83–8.96)	32.1 (NR)	31.7 (26–38)
		GP	312/262	8.2 (7.09–9.46)	33.0 (NR)	38.4 (32–44)
		PCb	308/261	7.9 (6.86–8.86)	33.0 (NR)	36.8 (31–43)
Treat, 2010[59]	1135	GCb	379/356	7.9 (7.1-9.2) p=0.693	33.9 (29.1-38.7)	96 (21.0-30.0)
		GP	377/355	8.5 (7.6-10.0)	36.2 (31.3-41.1)	121 (27.4-37.1)
		PCb	379/366	8.7 (7.7-9.9)	35.6 (30.7-40.4)	113 (25.3-34.7)
Kosmidis[72]	512/ 452	PG	219	9.97 (8.74-12.0)	42	31(25.12-37.60)
		GCb	219	10.49 (9.04-11.94)	42	27 (21.63-33.60)
Hsu[71]	85/ 80	GC	41	13.2 (10.4-16.0)	54.8	31.0 (16.4-45.5)
		GEp	39	21.5 (9.4-33.6)	74.4	37.2 (22.2-52.3)

*New entries are shaded.
$^a N_{eval}$ only reported when analysis was not intention-to-treat.
Cb, carboplatin; CI, confidence interval; D, docetaxel; G, gemcitabine; N_{eval}, number of patients evaluable; N_{rand}, number of patients randomized; NR, not reported; P, paclitaxel; V, vinorelbine; Ep, epirubicin

Summary of Key Sub-question 1.4

New trials continue to support the conclusion by the CCO that doublet chemotherapy including a platinum agent probably has a slight advantage over nonplatinum doublets (GRADE=moderate).

Key Sub-question 1.5. Are new doublets containing cisplatin more effective than doublets containing carboplatin?

The review by the CCO identified three relevant meta-analyses.[73-75] In the meta-analysis by Jiang et al., they found a higher overall response rate with cisplatin-based regimens when added to new drugs (RR 0.87;0.78-0.97, P=0.01) and when added to the same drug (RR 0.79; 0.70-0.89; P=0.0001) without a corresponding improvement in 1-year survival (RR 0.98; 0.90-1.07; P=0.66- new agent) (RR, 0.91;0.82-1.01; P=0.07).[75] The meta-analysis by Hotta et al. found superior survival with platinum-based combinations containing cisplatin over those containing carboplatin plus the same agent (HR= 1.106; 95% CI: 1.005-1.218; P=0.039).[74] It also found a greater objective response rate when using cisplatin over carboplatin (OR= 1.38; 95% CI: 1.14-1.67; P=0.001). In the meta-analysis by Ardizzoni et al, there was a greater mortality risk in those treated with carboplatin compared to those treated with cisplatin in patients with nonsquamous histology (HR=1.12; 95% CI: 1.01-1.23).[73]

Literature Relevant to this Sub-question Not Included in the CCO Review

We found one additional trial.[64] It compared vinorelbine plus cisplatin and paclitaxel plus carboplatin finding no significant difference between the two regimens in median survival 8.1 (6.7-9.6) months for the cisplatin containing regimen compared to 8.6 (7.2-10.7) for the carboplatin containing regimen. The overall response rates were 28 and 25%, respectively. However, the difference in second agents in the doublet precludes reaching a conclusion about differences between carboplatin and cisplatin.

Summary of Key Sub-question 1.5

One new trial does not alter the conclusion by the CCO that cisplatin combinations may have a slight advantage over carboplatin combinations in terms of survival and response rate. However, carboplatin generally has a milder toxicity than cisplatin (GRADE=moderate).

Key Sub-question 1.6. Does triplet chemotherapy consisting of a platinum agent plus a new agent improve clinical outcomes compared with doublet chemotherapy consisting of a platinum agent plus a new agent?

The review by the CCO identified updated guidelines published by the ACCP in 2007 which contained a meta-analysis of 28 trials and 12 additional RCTs where the addition of a third chemotherapeutic agent failed to show superiority over conventional doublets.[76] Though they found that response rates did improve, this was at the cost of substantially increased toxicity with the triplets, leading to a recommendation of the two-drug combination. In addition to the trials analyzed for the ACCP guidelines, the CCO found six additional trials investigating triplet regimens, none of which found a difference in median or 1-year survival with toxicity generally more frequent with the triplet regimens.[77-82]

New Literature Since 2007 Relevant to this Sub-question

We identified a systematic review not in the review by the CCO that was relevant to this question.[24] Azim and colleagues identified six trials including 1,932 patients who received either third generation triplet therapy or standard doublet therapy. Pooled analyses showed that triplet therapy resulted in a statistically significant increase in response rate (pooled OR=1.33, 95%

CI: 1.50-2.23), however overall survival was improved by less than six weeks (42.8 vs. 37.4 weeks) and this was not statistically significant. Patients receiving triplet therapy had statistically significantly more grade III/IV toxicities than patients receiving doublet therapy. The authors concluded that triplet therapy "is associated with higher tumor response rate at the expense of increased toxicity."[24]

We found four new trials,[83, 84] one of which was included in the review by Azim and colleagues.[84] The first trial randomized 433 patients into 4 arms of treatment- gemcitabine-cisplatin, gemcitabine-vinorelbine, gemcitabine-ifosfamide-cisplatin or gemcitabine-ifosfamide-vinorelbine.[83] They found no benefit with the addition of ifosfamide to a gemcitabine based doublet. Overall survival was 10.4 (9.4-12.2) months for the doublet and 10.3 (9.2-11.8) months for the triplet and the response rate was 29% (23-35) for the doublet and 26% (21-33) for the triplet. The second trial had 433 patients randomly assigned to gemcitabine-vinorelbine, gemcitabine-paclitaxel, gemcitabine-vinorelbine-cisplatin, gemcitabine-paclitaxel-cisplatin.[84] They found an increase in the response rate with triplets over doublets, 48% (42-54) vs. 35% (32-38). However, there was no benefit in overall survival with triplets having a median OS of 10.7 months and doublets having an overall survival of 10.5 months (P=0.379).

We also found one trial that compared a platinum-based triplet (paclitaxel, carboplatin, gemcitabine) versus a nonplatinum doublet (gemcitabine + vinorelbine). There were no statistically significant differences in overall survival between groups (10.7 vs. 10.3 months), and certain toxicities were greater in the triplet therapy group.[85] Another "triplet vs. doublet" study compared a nonplatinum triplet (vinorelbine, gemcitabine, docetaxel) to carboplatin plus paclitaxel and showed no statistically significantly difference in overall survival (13.6 vs. 14.1 months), with toxicity greater in the platinum doublet treated patients.[86]

Summary of Key Sub-question 1.6

New trials continue to support the conclusion by the CCO that triplet cytotoxic therapy might have some slight advantages in terms of response rate but at an increased risk of toxicity (GRADE=high).

Key Sub-question 1.7. Does the addition of targeted therapy to doublet chemotherapy consisting of a platinum agent plus a new agent improve outcomes compared with doublet chemotherapy consisting of a platinum agent and a new agent?

The review by the CCO identified eight trials of adding targeted therapy to conventional chemotherapy. They found that aprinocarsen did not improve outcomes in patients with advanced disease. Four trials of the tyrosine kinase inhibitors (TKI) failed to show an improvement in survival or response. However erlotinib was shown to significantly increase survival when a particular subgroup of 116 patients, who had never smoked, received the drug. When combined with paclitaxel and carboplatin, this subgroup had a median survival of 22.5 months compared with 10.1 months for placebo patients (P=0.01). In another subgroup study of only 18 patients, the Tarceva Lung Cancer Investigation trial, erlotinib led to significantly longer progression-free survival compared to placebo (7.9 months versus 5.4 months, P=0.02). Two of the trials looked at addition of bevacizumab. The first added bevacizumab to paclitaxel and carboplatin in a population restricted to those with Eastern Cooperative Oncology Group (ECOG) performance scores of 0-1, no brain metastases, nonsquamous cell histology, no hemoptysis and no history of bleeding diathesis or coagulopathy. In these 878 patients median survival increased by 2 months in the bevacizumab group (12.3 versus 10.3 months, HR= 0.79, 95% CI: 0.67-0.92; P=0.003) in addition to an improvement in response rate (35 vs. 15%, P<0.001). The second trial added bevacizumab to gemcitabine and cisplatin and found some improvement in response and a very modest improvement in progression-free survival, but no difference in overall survival. There were two trials adding cetuximab. The first added cetuximab to cisplatin and vinorelbine in 1125 patients whose tumors were immunohistochemically positive for epidermal growth factor receptor (EGFR) expression. There was improved survival with cetuximab (HR=0.871; 95% CI: 0.762-0.996; median 11.3 vs. 10.1 months). Response rates were also improved with cetuximab (36 vs. 29%, P=0.01). The other trial, which added cetuximab to carboplatin and taxane, did not show improvement in survival, or progression-free survival.

New Literature Since 2007 Relevant to this Sub-question

Our update search identified an additional 10 trials relevant to this sub-question.[87-96] Details of these trials, in addition to the eight contained in the review by the CCO, are presented in Table F4. Two of the new trials were of the agent PF-3512676. The first of these two trials, of 839 patients, did not find an improvement in OS or PFS and, in fact was halted based on efficacy, futility, and increased toxicity.[92] The other study of this agent had similar findings in 828 patients and was therefore also halted.[90] There was one study of endostar which enrolled 126 patients and found improvement in the overall response rate of 39.3% in the treatment group versus 23.0% in the control group (p=0.078).[89] However, there was no significant difference in the overall survival (17.6 vs. 15.8 months, p=0.696). There were two reports of bevacizumab. One of these had 1043 patients and was included in the review by the CCO,[95] and the other was the Asian subset of that population, consisting of 105 patients.[93] In the overall sample, as noted above, an improvement in progression-free survival was found. However this did not translate into an improvement in overall survival, which was about 13 months in each group.[95] In the study of the Asian subset, however, bevacizumab at a dose of 7.5 mg/kg improved the overall survival in Asian patients compared to placebo (HR=0.46, 95% CI: 0.22-0.97).[93] The other agents failed to show positive results. One trial of sorafenib found no clinical benefit and, in fact, was halted after an interim analysis found higher mortality in patients with squamous cell histology taking sorafenib than those in the placebo group.[96] Another study that was halted examined cediranib.[88] That trial was halted to review imbalances in assigned causes of death. A trial of cetuximab found a slight improvement in overall survival but this was not statistically significant, 9.69 months with cetuximab vs. 8.38 months with standard chemotherapy alone, (HR= 0.890, 95% CI: 0.754-1.051; p=.169).[91] There were two trials of bexarotene with chemotherapy.[87, 94] The first looked at 612 patients and found little difference in overall survival (8.5 vs. 9.2 months) or overall response (19.3 vs. 23.5%, p=.24).[87] However, when they examined a subpopulation of those with hypertriglyceridemia, they found that those with hypertriglyceridemia had significantly longer median survival than control patients (12.4 vs. 9.2 months; log-rank, P=.014). The other trial was of 623 patients and found the same, no significant difference (OS: 8.7 vs. 9.9 months, P=.3, ORR: 16.7 vs. 24.4%, P=.0224) except in those with hypertriglyceridemia (OS 12.3 months).[94] As both of these results were post-hoc subgroup analyses, their results should be interpreted with caution.

Table F4. Targeted Agents (adapted from Goffin)

Study Reference	N_{rand}/N_{eval}[a]	Comparison Agents	N_{rand}/N_{eval}[a]	Survival (95% CI), p Value Median (mo)	1-yr %	Overall Response (95% CI), p Value
Gatzemeier et al.[97]	1172/1159	EGC GC	580 579	9.9 (NR) 10.1 (NR)	41 (NR) 42 (NR)	31.5 29.9
Giaccone et al.[98]	1093/—	GCGe$_{500 mg/d}$ GCGe$_{250 mg/d}$ GC	365 365 363	9.9 (NR) p = 0.4560[b] 9.9 (NR) 10.9 (NR)	43 (NR) 41 (NR) 44 (NR)	50.3 (NR) ps = ns 51.2 (NR) 47.2 (NR)
Herbst et al.[99]	1079/—	PECb PCb	539 540	10.6 (NR) 10.5 (NR)	46.9 (NR)[c] 43.8 (NR)	21.5 (NR) p = 0.36 19.3 (NR)
Herbst et al.[100]	1037/—	PG e$_{500 mg/d}$Cb PG e$_{250 mg/d}$Cb PCb	347 345 345	8.7 (NR) 9.8 (NR) 9.9 (NR)	37 (NR) p = 0.64[a] 41 (NR) 42 (NR)	30.0 (NR) ps = ns 30.4 (NR) 28.7 (NR)
Sandler et al.[101]	878/850	PCb PCb + B	444/433 434/417	10.3 (NR)[d] 12.3 (NR)	44 (NR) 51 (NR)	15 (NR) p < 0.001 35 (NR)
Reck et al.[102]	1043/—	GC GC + B$_{7.5 mg/kg}$ GC + B$_{15 mg/kg}$	347 345 351	6.1 NR 6.7 NR 6.5 NR	NR NR NR	20 (NR) 34 (NR) 30 (NR)
Paz-Ares et al.[103]	670/—	GC GC + Ap	328 342	10.4 (8.6-12.2) 10.0 (8.4-10.8)	44.9 (NR)[e] 41.8 (NR)	35.0 (NR) p = 0.12 28.9 (NR)
Pirker et al.[104]	1125/—	C + V + Ce C + V	557 568	11.3 (0.762) p = 0.044 10.1 (0.996)	47 (NR) 42 (NR)	36 p = 0.010 29 (NR)
Manegold[92]	839	GC+PF-3512676 GC	416 423	11.0, p=0.98 10.7	47.0 45.7	32.2 31
Gaafar[105]	173	Ge Pl	86 87	10.9,(0.60-1.15) p=0.2 9.4	NR NR	NR NR
Hirsh[90]	828	PCb+PF-3512676 PCb	408 420	10.0 (0.81-1.12), p=.56 9.8	40.4,p=.73 41.6	28,p=.08 23
Han[89]	126	PCb+ ES PCb + Pl	63 63	17.6(13.4-21.7) p=0.696 15.8(9.4-22.9)	61.7, p=0.462 55.1	39.3, p=0.078 23.0
Mok[93] Asian subset of Reck, below	1043/105	GC+B7.5mg GC+B15mg GC+Pl	38 34 33	improved, but no details	NR	48.5 27.6 10.3
Reck, 2009[95]	1043	GC+B7.5mg GC+B15mg GC+Pl	345 351 347	13.6(0.86-1.23) p=0.761 13.4 13.1 (0.78-1.11) p=0.420	NR	37.8,p<.0001 34.6,p<0.0002 21.6
Scagliotti[96]	926	PCb+S PCb	464 462	10.7 (9.1-13.9) 10.6 (9.6-12.0)	terminated when analysis concluded study unlikely to reach endpoint	
Lynch[91]	676	Ct+TxCb TxCb	338 338	9.69(0.754-1.051) p=.1685 8.38	NR	25.7 (21.2-30.7) p=.0066 17.2 (13.3-21.6)
Takeda[106]	604/603	Platinum doublet chemotherapy Ge (after 3 cycles of chemotherapy)	301 302	12.9 (0.72-1.03), p=.11 13.7	NR	29.3,p=.20 34.2
Goss[88]	296/251	PCb+Pl PCb + Cd	126 125	study halted to review imbalances in assigned causes of death	NR	38,p<.0001 16
Blumenschein[87]	612	BxCbP CbP	306 306	8.5 9.2	NR	19.3,p=.24 23.5
Ramlau[94]	623	CV CVBx	312 311	9.9,p=.3 8.7	NR	24.4,p=.0224 16.7

*New entries are shaded.
[a] N_{eval} only reported when analysis was not intention-to-treat.
[b] Log rank comparison of three arms.
[c] Hazard ratio of overall survival for PECb vs. PCb was 0.995 (0.86 –1.16), p = 0.95.
[d] HR for death = 0.79 (0.67– 0.92), p = 0.003.
[e] Hazard ratio of overall survival for GC vs. GC = Ap was 1.05 (0.88 –1.25), p = 0.61.
Ap, aprinocarsen; B, bevacizumab; C, cisplatin; Cb, carboplatin; Ce, cetuximab; CI, confidence interval; E, erlotinib; G, gemcitabine; Ge, gefitinib; N_{eval}, number of patients evaluable; N_{rand}, number of patients randomized; NR, not reported; P, paclitaxel; V, Vinorelbine; Pl, placebo; ES, endostar; S, sorafenib; Ct, cetuximab; Tx, taxane; Cd, cediranib; Bx, bexarotene

Key Sub-question 1.7.1 Does targeted monotherapy improve outcomes in selected patient populations?

We also identified seven publications (from six trials) that assessed the use of targeted monotherapy compared to conventional chemotherapy, primarily in the population of patients with the EGFR gene mutation. We consider this to be related but distinct to the above discussion regarding the addition of targeted therapy to conventional chemotherapy, and therefore have created a new key sub-question for this topic. These studies, which compared gefitinib to carboplatin-paclitaxel in a general population and then performed a subgroup analysis on patients with the EGFR mutation,[107, 108] gefitinib vs. chemotherapy in patients selected for EGFR gene mutations,[109, 110] gefitinib vs. chemotherapy in a general population and then performed a subgroup analysis on patients with EGFR mutations,[111] and erlotinib vs. chemotherapy in patients selected for EGFR gene mutations,[112, 113] consistently show large differences in progression-free survival favoring targeted monotherapy, such as 10.1 months vs. 5.4 months(Table F5). Overall survival also tended to favor groups treated with targeted monotherapy as opposed to chemotherapy treatment, but this has not reached statistical significance, and two trials favored chemotherapy over targeted monotherapy, however neither of these contradictory findings reached statistically significance either.[111, 113] One of these trials was consistent with the support for targeted monotherapy compared to chemotherapy within a subgroup analysis of patients with EGFR mutations.[111] Other than rash and aminotransferase elevation, erlotinib and gefitinib were also in general better tolerated than cytotoxic chemotherapy.

Table F5. Targeted Monotherapy

Study Reference	N_{rand}/N_{eval}^a	Comparison Agents	N_{rand}/N_{eval}^a	Progression Free Survival (95% CI), p Value	Overall Response (95% CI), p Value
Mok, 2009[108]	1217/1177	Ge CbP	609/597 608/550	Hazard ratio favoring treatment with gefitinib = 0.74 (95% CI 0.65-0.85)	Hazard ratio favoring treatment with gefitinib = 0.91 (95% CI, 0.76-1.10)
Maemondo, 2010[109] All patients had EGFR mutations	230/224	Ge CbP	115/114 115/110	Hazard ratio favoring treatment with gefitinib = 0.30, 95% CI (0.22-0.41)	2 year survival Ge 61.4% CbP 46.7% (p=0.31)
Mitsudomi, 2010[110] All patients had EGFR mutations	177/172	Ge CD	86/88 86/89	Hazard ratio favoring treatment with gefitinib = 0.49 (95% CI 0.34-0.71), p=0.0001	Hazard ratio favoring treatment with gefitinib = 0.61 (95% CI 0.28-1.34)
Zhou, 2011[112] All patients had EGFR mutations	165/154	E CbP	83/82 82/72	Hazard ratio favoring treatment with erlotinib = 0.16 (95% CI 0.10-0.26)	NR
Han, 2012[111] Total population	313/309	Ge GC	309/159 309/150	Hazard ratio favoring treatment with gefitinib = 0.83 (95% CI 0.66-1.06), p=0.138	Hazard ratio showed no clinically important difference: 1.07 (95% CI 0.82-1.40), p=.604
EGFR mutation subgroup	--/96	Ge GC	--/53 --/43	Hazard ratio favoring treatment with gefitinib = 0.544 (95% CI 0.27-1.10)	Hazard ratio showed no clinically important difference: 0.96 (95% CI 0.46-2.00)
Rosell, 2012[113] All patients had EGFR mutations	173/173	E CD or CG	86/86 87/87	Hazard ratio favoring treatment with erlotinib = 0.37 (95% CI 0.25-0.54), p<0.0001	ratio showed no clinically important difference: 1.04 (95% CI 0.65-1.67), p=0.87

$^a N_{eval}$ only reported when analysis was not intention-to-treat.
Ge, gefitinib; Cb, carboplatin; P, paclitaxel; E, erlotinib; C, cisplatin; D, Docetaxel; G, gemcitabine

One additional trial is relevant to this topic. Gridelli and colleagues compared a strategy of using erlotinib as first-line therapy in unselected patients with advanced NSCLC, followed by cisplatin and gemcitabine at the first sign of progression, versus the opposite strategy of initial therapy of cisplatin and gemcitabine followed by erlotinib given at the first sign of progression.[114] Among nearly 800 patients, the erlotinib first strategy was significantly worse in terms of overall survival.

As part of an update search, we identified two recently published meta-analyses of tyrosine kinase inhibitors.[13, 22] One meta-analysis was of monotherapy with either erlotinib or gefitinib compared to cytotoxic therapy in patients with advanced NSCLC and EGFR mutations.[13] It included six trials, all of which are included in Table F5. The pooled analysis showed a statistically significant benefit for progression-free survival (HR=0.37; 95% CI: 0.27-0.52), and a nonstatistically significant benefit in overall survival (HR=0.94; 95%CI: 0.77-1.15). The second meta-analysis was restricted to gefitinib, and included studies of it as monotherapy, combined with systemic chemotherapy, and then given after systemic chemotherapy (only one trial of this).[22] The monotherapy portion included four trials, three of which are included in Table F5, and also found improvement in progression-free survival for patients with EGFR mutations.

Summary of Key Sub-question 1.7

New trials of a number of novel targeted agents have so far failed to find results equivalent to the increases in progression-free survival seen with erlotinib (mostly in patients who have never smoked) and bevacizumab (in an Asian population subgroup analysis) in the CCO review (GRADE=moderate).

Erlotinib or gefitinib monotherapy is in general superior in terms of beneficial outcomes and adverse events than cytotoxic chemotherapy in patients with EGFR mutations (GRADE=high).

Key Sub-question 1.8. Is a single new agent superior to best supportive care?

We did not update this key sub-question as our scope was the comparative effectiveness between drugs.

Key Sub-question 1.9. Is a single new agent superior to single-agent or doublet therapy including older agents?

The CCO review focused on cytotoxic "new agents" such as vinorelbine and irinotecan and not targeted therapies. As an earlier conclusion had already established doublet therapy as the treatment of choice, we did not update this key sub-question.

Key Sub-question 1.10. Which single new agent is most effective?

The CCO review focused on the single agent cytotoxic agents gemcitabine, vinorelbine, paclitaxel, and docetaxel. Since an earlier conclusion had established doublet therapy as the treatment of choice, we did not update this key sub-question.

Key Sub-question 1.11. What is the optimal administration, duration, and timing of chemotherapy for advanced NSCLC?

We did not update this key sub-question as it did not assess comparative effectiveness of agents and therefore did not fit the scope of key question #1 for this current review.

Key Sub-question 1.12. Is a Doublet Regimen Better than a Single Agent for the Elderly Population?

In the systematic review by the CCO, six trials were identified as being relevant to the treatment of elderly patients with NSCLC.[2] These trials compared a variety of different regimens, including singlet vs. singlet, singlet vs. doublet, and singlet vs. best supportive care. The CCO original key question was refined by our TEP to focus solely on singlet vs. doublet therapy in elderly patients. Four trials in the CCO review compared singlet versus doublet therapy. Two of the trials reported modestly improved overall survival in the doublet-treated patients, and the other two reported no differences. The CCO review concluded that using a single new agent was superior to best supportive care in patients > 70 years of age; doublet therapy could be considered in those that could tolerate combination therapy or platinum agents; and that no trial that had been dedicated to assessing platinum agents in the elderly population has been completed. For patients > 70 years, survival was similar to that in younger patients, even though the elderly experienced more frequent leucopenia. There was a lack of data regarding the use of chemotherapy in patients >80 years of age and, therefore, chemotherapy should be used cautiously in that population.

New Literature Since 2007 Relevant to this Sub-question

We identified four new trials that compared single agents to doublet regimens in the elderly population.[108, 113, 115, 116] The first two trials were focused on elderly patients.[108, 113] The second two trials examined the elderly as a subpopulation.[115, 116]

The first trial focused specifically on the elderly population, comparing treatment with docetaxel to treatment with both docetaxel and gemcitabine.[116] Three hundred and fifty patients were randomized, with the median age of 74 years. ITT analysis showed median survival of 5.5 months in the group receiving the doublet chemotherapy, compared to 5.1 months in those receiving a single agent (P=.65). The median time-to-progression was longer in those receiving the doublet regimen (4.8 months) compared to those receiving a single agent (2.9 months; P=.004).

The second trial compared individuals aged 70-89 receiving either the doublet regimen of carboplatin and paclitaxel or therapy with a single agent of vinorelbine or gemcitabine.[115] The 451 patients were randomly assigned to the two groups. Median overall survival was 10.3 months for the doublet chemotherapy compared to 6.2 months for therapy with a single agent (HR 0.64, 95% CI 0.52-0.78; p<0.0001). One year survival was also greater in the doublet group with 44.5% (95% CI 37.9-50.9) alive at one year compared to 25.5% in the single agent group (95% CI 19.9-31.3). There were greater toxic effects in the doublet chemotherapy group but this was still considered a superior regimen to single agent therapy.

The first subgroup trial assessed elderly patients within a group of adults treated for NSCLC compared erlotinib to standard chemotherapy of cisplatin or carboplatin plus docetaxel or gemcitabine.[113] The study was halted after interim analysis revealed that the study had met its primary endpoint. In the final analysis, the median progression-free survival for those treated with erlotinib was 9.7 months (95% CI 8.4-12.3) compared to 5.2 months for those treated with the doublet regimen (95% CI 4.5-5.8) (HR 0.37, 95% CI 0.25-0.54; p<0.0001). A multivariable analysis of progression-free survival found that age was not a significant factor.

Another subgroup study assessed differences in progression-free survival in patients treated with gefitinib compared to carboplatin plus paclitaxel.[108] They found that progression-free survival was longer in the gefitinib group but that this was affected by age. For those patients younger than 65, the hazard ratio was 0.81; 95% CI, 0.70 - 0.95, and for those patients 65 years or older, the hazard ratio was 0.58; 95% CI, 0.45-0.76; P<0.001. There was a statistically significant interaction between age and treatment effect (p=0.03).

We add here one additional trial, which compared singlet vs. doublet therapy, although the mean age of patients was "elderly" (mean age = 63), and not all clinical experts would judge this study as relevant to the elderly population.[117] This study compared docetaxel alone to docetaxel plus gemcitabine in 312 patients with stage IIIB or IV NSCLC. There was a slight, statistically significant advantage for overall survival in the doublet-treated group (9.4 months vs. 8.3 months). There was a greater proportion of patients in the doublet-treated group with grade 2-4 anemia, plus two treatment-related deaths.

Summary of Key Sub-question 1.12

With the exception of studies of gefitinib and erlotinib monotherapy (in patients with EGFR mutations), doublet chemotherapy probably has a slight benefit in terms of survival compared to singlet therapy, but causes more toxicity (GRADE=moderate). Also, there now has been one trial of platinum therapy in the elderly taken to completion that found a near-doubling of the proportion of patients alive at one year in the doublet therapy group compared to monotherapy.

Key Sub-question 1.13. Toxicity of first-line systemic chemotherapy regimens

The CCO reported a summary of Grade 3 or 4 chemotherapy toxicities from 7 large trials of various agents. They cautioned that "comparisons between trials should be avoided and numbers are provided only to give a general sense of the toxicity of the regimens," which we now repeat. To the table from the CCO we have added the Grade 3 or 4 toxicities from additional large trials of first line treatment, see Table F6.

Table F6. Summary of Grade 3 or 4 Chemotherapy Toxicity (% Patients) from Large, Selected Trials in NSCLC (adapted from Goffin)

Regimen Dose (mg/m²) and Administration Schedule [Reference]	Febrile Neutropenia	Anemia	Nausea/ Vomiting	Peripheral Neuropathy	Platelets	Renal
Paclitaxel 100 over 1 hr days 1, 8, 15 every 4 weeks [Comella 2004[118]]	3	2	NR/0	0	0	0
Gemcitabine 1200 over 30 mins days 1, 8, 15 every 4 weeks [Comella 2004 [118]]	3	10	NR/3	2	10	2
Vinorelbine 30 days 1, 8 every 3 weeks [Gridelli 2003[119]]	NR	<4	<1	1	<1	0
Docetaxel 60 over 1hr, day 1 every 3 weeks [Kudoh 2006[120]]	12.5	3.4	10.2	0	0	NR
Cisplatin/Vinorelbine 100 day 1/25 days 1, 8, 15, 22 every 4 weeks [Fossella 2003[50]]	5	24	16/16	4 (Sensory)	4	NR
Cisplatin/Vinorelbine 80 day 8/30 days 1 and 8 [Georgoulias 2005[121]]	NR	6	15‡	NR	6	3
Cisplatin/Paclitaxel 75 day 2/135 (24 hour) day 1 every 3 weeks [Schiller 2002[45]]	16	13	25/24	5	6	3*
Cisplatin/Docetaxel 75 day 1/75 day 1 every 3 weeks [Fossella 2003[50]]	5	7#	10/8	4 (Sensory)	3	NR
Cisplatin/Docetaxel 75 day 1/75 day 1 every 3 weeks [Schiller 2002[45]]	11	15	24/21	5	3	3*

Regimen Dose (mg/m²) and Administration Schedule [Reference]	Febrile Neutropenia	Anemia	Nausea/ Vomiting	Peripheral Neuropathy	Platelets	Renal
Cisplatin/Gemcitabine 100 day 1/1000 days 1, 8, 15 every 4 weeks [Schiller 2002[45]]	4†	28†	37/35	9	50†	9*†
Carboplatin/Paclitaxel AUC 6 day 1/225 (3 hour) day 1 every 3 weeks [Schiller 2002[45]]	4†	10	9†/8†	10	10	1*
Carboplatin/Paclitaxel AUC 6 day 1/200 (3 hour) day 1 every 3 weeks [Kosmidis 2002[122]]	1	5	4	8	2	0
Carboplatin/Docetaxel AUC 6 day 1/75 day 1 every 3 weeks [Fossella 2003[50]]	4	10#	6/4#	1 (Sensory)	7	NR
Gemcitabine/Docetaxel 1000 days 1 and 8/100 day 8 [Georgoulias 2005[121]]	NR	2	2‡	NR	4	0
Gemcitabine/Paclitaxel 1000 day 1, 8/200 (3 hour) day 1 every 3 weeks [Kosmidis 2002[122]]	2	2	7	6	1	1
Carboplatin/Paclitaxel AUC=6; 200 mg/m² [Sandler 2006[101]]	1.8	0.9	NR	NR	0.2	NR
Carboplatin/Paclitaxel/Bevacizumab AUC=6; 200 mg/m² 15 mg/kg/daily [Sandler 2006[101]]	4.0	0	NR	NR	1.6	NR
Cisplatin/Gemcitabine [Reck 2009[102]]	NR	13	4	NR	23	NR
Cisplatin/gemcitabine/ bevacizumab 4.5 mg/kg [Reck 2009[102]]	NR	10	7	NR	27	NR
Cisplatin/gemcitabine/bevacizumab 15 mg/kg [Reck 2009[102]]	NR	10	9	NR	23	NR

New entries are shaded.
Abbreviations: AUC = area under curve; hr = hour; mg=milligrams; m²= meters squared; min = minutes; NR = not reported; NSCLC = non-small cell lung cancer.
*Grades 3, 4, and 5 renal toxicity.
† Toxicity was significantly different than for the trial comparator regimen, cisplatin-paclitaxel (p=0.05).[Schiller 2002]
‡ Toxicity was significantly different between the two regimens, gemcitabine-docetaxel and cisplatin-vinorelbine (p<0.001).[Georgoulias 2005]
# Toxicity was significantly different than for the trial comparator regimen, cisplatin-vinorelbine (p<0.01). [Fossella 2003]

KEY QUESTION 2. For patients with metastatic NSCLC what is the comparative effectiveness of the different recommended (e.g. NCCN guidelines) second line chemotherapy regimens?

"Second-line therapy," by definition in this review, means active therapy. It has already been established that docetaxel monotherapy resulted in improved overall survival when compared to best supportive care. For example, more than a decade ago Shepherd and colleagues randomized 104 patients to either docetaxel at 75mg/m2 or 100mg/m2 or best supportive care (BSC).[123] The median overall survival was longer in the docetaxel groups with 7.0 months compared to the 4.6 months in the BSC group. The difference was more significant when comparing the docetaxel 75mg/m2 to the BSC with the median survival of 7.5 months compared to the 4.6 months of BSC (P=.010) One-year survival was also increased in the docetaxel 75mg/m2 group with 37% versus 11% in the BSC group (p=.003).

There was no single systematic review of second-line therapy that was both comprehensive and high quality, thus we found no equivalent to the review by the CCO. Therefore our synthesis of the second-line therapy first discusses the existing systematic reviews, and then the trials.

Existing Systematic Reviews

There were seven systematic reviews, details of which can be found in Table S1.

The first three reviews were done by Qi and colleagues.[124-126] The first of these consisted of five RCTs comparing pemetrexed doublets versus pemetrexed alone.[124] The two other trials by Qi and colleagues included drugs that do not have FDA approval (enzastaurin and matuximab).[125,126] Futhermore, the authors pooled data across studies that included a very heterogeneous group of drugs, including cytotoxic therapies and targeted therapies. We did not judge this pooling to be clinically sensible and hence concluded this meta-analysis was not relevant to clinical practice. Similarly, the second review by Qi and colleagues assesses the efficacy of vandetanib in a pooled analysis of heterogeneous comparators, and we likewise did not judge this as clinically meaningful.[125]

The third review consisted of eight RCTs comparing docetaxel- based doublets with docetaxel as a single agent.[126] These trials resulted in 2,126 patients for analysis. Meta-analysis showed no difference in overall survival (HR=0.93; 95% CI: 0.80-1.07, P=0.308) but did show a difference in overall response rate (OR=1.42, 95% CI: 1.13-1.80, P=0.03). In addition, 1-year survival was not significantly improved (OR=1.09, 95% CI: 0.92-1.28, P=0.328).

The next review was by Yang and colleagues and included four RCTs.[127] Two of these compared bevacizumab plus carboplatin and paclitaxel to carboplatin plus paclitaxel alone, one compared bevacizumab with chemotherapy to bevacizumab with erlotinib or chemotherapy alone, and the last compared cisplatin plus gemcitabine with either placebo or bevacizumab. Only one of these trials studied treatment exclusively as second-line therapy,[128] one trial included both untreated and recurrent nonsquamous cell disease,[102] and the other two studied bevacizumab as part of first line treatment.[101,129] These four studies combined treated 2101 patients. Meta-analysis found that tumor response rate might not be increased with low-dose bevacizumab (7.5mg/kg) (RR= 1.19, p=0.68) but was with high-dose treatment (15mg/kg) (RR=1.69, p=0.002). The one year survival rate was not increased with either low (RR=1.02, p=0.82) or high doses (RR=1.09, p=0.07). The 2 year survival rate was increased by the higher dose regimen but at a cost of greater toxicity. In the one study of bevacizumab as part of second line treatment,[128] the addition of bevacizumab to second line treatment with docetaxel or pemetrexed resulted in improvements in progression-free survival and overall survival, with hazard ratios of 0.66 to 0.78, although these improvements were not statistically significant. In this study, adding erlotinib to the bevacizumab therapy did not result in additional improvement. No study demonstrated that continuing bevacizumab beyond first line chemotherapy, either alone or with another agent, offers superior overall survival to stopping bevacizumab at the time of discontinuation of first line cytotoxic therapy.

The fifth systematic review by Mountzios and colleages included four trials of erlotinib versus placebo, erlotinib and gemcitabine-cisplatin, erlotinib and carboplatin-paclitaxel, and erlotinib and bevacizumab.[20] This review covered the use of erlotinib as first line, second line, and maintenance therapy. Regarding second-line therapy, assessment of overall survival found a modest absolute gain of 2 months (overall survival of 6.7 months vs. 4.7 months, HR = 0.70, p < 0.001) in the BR.21 trial.[130] This led to FDA (11/2004) and EMA (10/2005) approval of erlotinib for the treatment of chemotherapy-resistant patients.

The final two systematic reviews were by Di Maio and colleagues. The first was an individual patient data meta-analysis of docetaxel administered weekly or once every three weeks as second-line therapy in patients with NSCLC.[131] A total of 865 patients were included, 81 percent were performance status 0 or 1, 91 percent had received platinum therapy. There was no difference in median survival (27.4 weeks vs. 26.1 weeks), and fewer episodes of severe and febrile neutropenia in patients receiving weekly docetaxel. The second systematic review included the data from six trials comparing single agent and doublet chemotherapy.[132] Overall survival was not significantly different with the median of 37.3 weeks with doublets and 34.7 weeks with single agent (P=.32). The response rate was 15.1% with the doublets and 7.3% with a single agent (P=.0004). There were more toxic effects from the doublet, compared to single agent therapy.

The conclusions from the seven systematic reviews can be summarized as:

- doublet second line cytotoxic therapy might offer slight benefits in progression-free survival and response rate, not overall survival, but at a cost of increased toxicity;
- erlotinib produces modest increases in overall survival; and
- in one phase II study, the addition of bevacizumab to second line treatment resulted in improvements in survival that were not statistically significant.

Treatment of Metastatic Non-Small Cell Lung Cancer

Table S1. Second Line Systematic Reviews Published Since 2010

Author (Year)	Search End Date	What was compared / Studies included: First Author, Year Title, Journal	Overall Survival	Progression-free Survival	Overall Response Rate	Adverse Events	Other Outcomes Reported	Conclusions per abstract:
Qi et al. (2012)[124]	May 2011	**Pemetrexed and something vs. pemetrexed alone** Chiappori, 2010 Phase II, double-blinded, randomized study of enzastaurin plus pemetrexed as second-line therapy in patients with advanced non-small cell lung cancer. J Thorac Oncol De Boer, 2011 Vandetanib plus pemetrexed for the second-line treatment of advanced non-small-cell lung cancer: a randomized, double-blind phase III trial. J Clin Oncol Scagliotti, 2010 A randomized phase II study of bortezomib and pemetrexed, in combination or alone, in patients with previously treated advanced non-small-cell lung cancer. Lung Cancer Schiller, 2010 Pemetrexed with or without matuzumab as second-line treatment for patients with stage IIIB/IV non-small cell lung cancer. J Thorac Oncol Smit, 2009 Randomized phase II and pharmacogenetic study of pemetrexed compared with pemetrexed plus carboplatin in pretreated patients with advanced non-small cell lung cancer. J Clin Oncol	X					Pemetrexed based doublet therapy didn't gain any benefit in survival but significantly improved progression free survival and overall response competed with single agent pemetrexed. More adverse events in doublet group.
Qi et al. (2011)[125]	2011	**Vandetanib vs. Pemetrexed, Erlotinib, Docetaxel** Herbst, 2010 Vandetanib plus docetaxel versus docetaxel as second-line treatment for patients with advanced non-small-cell lung cancer (ZODIAC): a double-blind, randomized, phase 3 trial. Lancet Oncol Natale, 2011 Phase III trial of vandetanib compared with erlotinib in patients with previously treated advanced non-small-cell lung cancer. J Clin Oncol De Boer, 2011 Vandetanib plus pemetrexed for the second-line treatment of advanced non-small-cell lung cancer: a randomized, double-blind phase III trial. J Clin Oncol Heymach, 2007 Randomized, placebo-controlled phase II study of vandetanib plus II study of vandetanib plus docetaxel in previously treated non-small-cell lung cancer. J Clin Oncol	X	X	X	X		Vandetanib offered a clinically meaningful and statistically significant improvement in progression free survival and overall response rate in patients with advanced NSCLC but did not benefit overall survival.
Qi et al. (2012)[126]	March 2011	**Docetaxel; single vs. doublet treatment** Herbst, 2010 Vandetanib plus docetaxel versus docetaxel as second-line treatment for patients with advanced non-small-cell lung cancer (ZODIAC): a double-blind, randomized, phase 3 trial. Lancet Oncol Heymach, 2007 Randomized, placebo-controlled phase II study of vandetanib plus docetaxel in previously treated non-small-cell lung cancer. J Clin Oncol Gebbia, 2009 Weekly docetaxel vs. docetaxel-based combination chemotherapy as second-line treatment of advanced non-small-cell lung cancer patients. The DISTAL-2 randomized trial. Lung Cancer Pectasides, 2005 Comparison of docetaxel and docetaxel-irinotecan combination as second-line chemotherapy in advanced non-small-cell lung cancer; a randomized phase II trial. Ann Oncol Takeda, 2009 Phase II trial of docetaxel plus gemcitabine versus docetaxel in second-line treatment for non-small-cell lung cancer: results of a Japan Clinical Oncology Group trial (JCOG0104). Ann Oncol Pallis, 2010 A randomized phase III study of the docetaxel/carboplatin combination versus docetaxel single-agent as second line treatment for patients with advanced/metastatic non-small cell lung cancer. BMC Cancer Wachters, 2005 A randomized phase II trial of docetaxel vs. docetaxel and irinotecan in patients with stage IIIb-IV non-small-cell lung cancer who failed first-line treatment. Br J Cancer Segawa, 2010 A randomized phase II study of a combination of docetaxel and S-1 versus docetaxel monotherapy in patients with non-small cell lung cancer previously treated with platinum-based chemotherapy: results of Okayama Lung Cancer Study Group (OLCSG) Trial 0503. J Thorac Oncol	X	X	X	X	1 year survival	Docetaxel-based doublet therapy did not gain any benefit in survival but significantly improved progression free survival and better overall response rate. However more grade 3/4 neutropenia, thrombocytopenia, and diarrhea were observed in the docetaxel-based doublet group.

Treatment of Metastatic Non-Small Cell Lung Cancer

Author (Year)	Search End Date	What was compared / Studies included: First Author, Year Title. Journal	Overall Survival	Progression-free Survival	Overall Response Rate	Adverse Events	Other Outcomes Reported	Conclusions per abstract:
Yang et al. (2010)[127]	March 2009	Bevacizumab vs. various other agents in first or second-line therapy Herbst, 2010 Phase II study of efficacy and safety of bevacizumab in comparison with chemotherapy or erlotinib compared with chemotherapy alone for treatment of recurrent or refractory non-small-cell lung cancer. J Clin Oncol Johnson, 2004 Randomized phase II trial comparing bevacizumab plus carboplatin and paclitaxel with carboplatin and paclitaxel alone in previously untreated locally advanced or metastatic non-small-cell lung cancer. J Clin Oncol Sandler,2006 Paclitaxel-carboplatin alone or with bevacizumab for non-small-cell lung cancer. N Engl J Med Reck, 2009 Phase III trial of cisplatin plus gemcitabine with either placebo or bevacizumab as first-line therapy for nonsquamous non-small-cell lung cancer: AVAiL. J Clin Oncol	X	X		X	1st year survival, 2nd year survival, tumor response rate, treatment-related deaths	Low-dose bevacizumab may significantly improve PFS in patients with unresectable NSCLC, whereas high-dose bevacizumab may increase 2-year overall survival rates, prolong PFS and improve tumor response rate but at the cost of higher treatment related death.
Mountzios et al. (2011)[20]	Feb 2010	Erlotinib vs. placebo; TALENT-erlotinib + platinum-based doublet (gemcitabine/cisplatin), TRIBUTE-erlotinib + carboplatin/paclitaxel), ATLAS-erlotinib + bevacizumab Shepherd, 2005 Erlotinib in previously treated non-small-cell lung cancer. N Engl J Med Perez-Soler, 2004 Determinants of tumor response and survival with erlotinib in patients with non-small-cell lung cancer. J Clin Oncol Herbst, 2007 Phase II study of efficacy and safety of bevacizumab in combination with chemotherapy or erlotinib compared with chemotherapy alone for treatment of recurrent or refractory non small-cell lung cancer. J Clin Oncol Hainsworth, 2008 A phase III, multicenter, placebo-controlled, double-blind, randomized, clinical trial to evaluate the efficacy of bevacizumab (Avastin) in combination with erlotinib (Tarceva) compared with erlotinib alone for treatment of advanced non-small cell lung cancer (NSCLC) after failure of standard first line chemotherapy (BETA). J Thorac Oncol	X	X	X	X	Risk of death	Despite the modest absolute gain in OS (2 months), the [Shepherd] study demonstrated a 30% reduction in the risk of death in this heavily pre-treated group of patients. On the basis of these results, erlotinib received both FDA and EMA approval in November 2004 and October 2005, respectively, for the treatment of chemotherapy-resistant patients with advanced NSCLC. Based on the results of the SATURN and ATLAS studies, the use of erlotinib as maintenance therapy is becoming a treatment option for patients with good performance status (PS) who respond to first-line chemotherapy.
Di Maio (2009)[132] Identified by TEP, predates 2010	June 2008	Single vs. Combination Takeda, 2009 Phase III trial of docetaxel plus gemcitabine versus docetaxel in second-line treatment for non-small-cell lung cancer: Results of a Japan Clinical Oncology Group trial (JCOG0104). Ann Oncol Georgoulias, 2004 Irinotecan plus gemcitabine vs. irinotecan for the second-line treatment of patients with advanced non-small-cell cancer pretreated with docetaxel and cisplatin: A multicentre, randomized, phase II study. Br J Cancer Georgoulias, 2005 Second-line treatment with irinotecan plus cisplatin vs. cisplatin of patients with advanced non-small-cell lung cancer pretreated with taxanes and gemcitabine: A multicenter randomized phase II study. Br J Cancer Wachters, 2005 A randomized phase II trial of docetaxel vs. docetaxel and irinotecan in patients with stage IIIb-IV non-small-cell lung cancer who failed first-line treatment. Br J Cancer Gebbia, 2009 Weekly docetaxel vs. docetaxel-based combination chemotherapy as second-line treatments of advanced non-small-cell lung cancer patients: The DISTAL-2 randomized trial. Lung Cancer Smit, 2008 A randomized phase II study of pemetrexed (P) versus pemetrexed-carboplatin (PC) as second line treatment for patients (pts) with advanced non-small-cell lung cancer (NSCLC)- NVALT 7. J Clin Oncol	X	X	X	X		Doublet chemotherapy as second-line treatment of advanced NSCLC significantly increases response rate and progression-free survival, but is more toxic and does not improve overall survival compared to single-agent.

Treatment of Metastatic Non-Small Cell Lung Cancer

Author (Year)	Search End Date	What was compared / Studies included: First Author, Year Title, Journal	Overall Survival	Progression-free Survival	Overall Response Rate	Adverse Events	Other Outcomes Reported	Conclusions per abstract:
Di Maio (2007)[131] Identified by peer review, predates 2010	December 2005	Docetaxel; Weekly vs. Once every three weeks						Weekly docetaxel shows similar efficacy compared to docetaxel administered once every three weeks, and represents an alternative for second line treatment of advanced NSCLC.
		Gridelli, 2004 A randomized clinical trial of two docetaxel regimens (weekly vs. 3 week) in the second-line treatment of non-small-cell lung cancer: The DISTAL 01 study. Br J Cancer						
		Gervais, 2005 Phase II randomized trial comparing docetaxel given every 3 weeks with weekly schedule as second-line therapy in patients with advanced non-small-cell lung cancer (NSCLC). Ann Oncol						
		Schuette, 2005 Phase III study of second-line chemotherapy for advanced non-small-cell lung cancer with weekly compared with 3-weekly docetaxel. J Clin Oncol						
		Lai, 2005 Phase II randomized trial of tri-weekly versus day 1 and 8 weekly docetaxel as a second-line treatment of advanced non-small cell lung cancer. Jpn J Clin Oncol						
		Camps, 2006 Randomized phase III study of 3-weekly versus weekly docetaxel in pretreated advanced non-small-cell lung cancer: A Spanish Lung Cancer Group trial. Ann Oncol	X		X	X		

Clinical Trials Published Since 2006

We identified 20 trials, six of which were also included in the systematic reviews above.[133-138] Table S2 shows the overlap between trials and systematic reviews.

Trials Included in Existing Systematic Reviews

Two of the trials, by Gebbia and colleagues[133] and Takeda and colleagues,[134] were included in the review by Di Maio and colleagues discussed previously.[132] One trial by Herbst and colleagues[136] was in the review by Yang and colleagues,[127] also discussed previously. The remaining three trials were only included in reviews by Qi and colleagues, which were not discussed in detail in the prior section. We therefore summarize these three trials here.

The first trial[135] was included in Qi and colleagues (2012).[126] In this RCT, patients who had been pretreated with front-line platinum-free regimens were randomized to receive either docetaxel-carboplatin or docetaxel alone. There was no significant difference in overall survival between the two groups with 10.27 (95% CI: 7.07-13.47) months achieved in the combination arm and 7.70 (95% CI: 3.39-12.01) months in the docetaxel alone arm (p=0.550). The response rate was similar 10.4% for the combination versus 7.7% (p=0.764). Likewise, the one-year survival rate was similar 43.8% versus 40.3%.

The next trial[137] was included in the systematic reviews by Qi and colleagues (2011)[125] and Qi and colleagues (2012).[124] In this study, 534 patients were randomized to receive vandetanib added to pemetrexed or pemetrexed plus placebo. There was no significant difference in overall survival. Median overall survival was 10.5 months for vandetanib and 9.2 months for placebo (HR=0.86; 97.54% CI, 0.65-1.13; p=.219). There were statistically significant improvements in overall response rate with 19% in the vandetanib group and 8% in the placebo group (p<.001). Vandetanib is not currently approved for use in the United States.

The last of the trials[138] was found in Qi and colleagues (2011).[125] In this trial 1,240 patients were randomized to receive vandetanib or erlotinib. There was no significant difference in the superiority analysis as the median overall survival was 6.9 months for vandetanib and 7.8 months with erlotinib (HR=1.01; p=.830). Likewise, the overall response rate was 12% in both arms (two-sided P=.98). A preplanned non-inferiority analysis supported non-inferiority, defined as whether vandetanib "retained at least 50%" of the efficacy of erlotinib.

Table S2. Second Line Trials Appearing in a Systematic Review

First Author, Year Title. Journal	Systematic Reviews Including this Trial*
Single versus Double	
Gebbia, 2009[133] Weekly docetaxel vs. docetaxel-based combination chemotherapy as second-line treatments of advanced non-small-cell lung cancer patients: The DISTAL-2 randomized trial. Lung Cancer	Di Maio (2009)[132] Qi (2012)[126]
Takeda, 2009[134] Phase III trial of docetaxel plus gemcitabine versus docetaxel in second-line treatment for non-small-cell lung cancer: Results of a Japan Clinical Oncology Group trial (JCOG0104). Ann Oncol	Di Maio (2009)[132] Qi (2012)[126]
Pallis, 2010[135] A randomized phase III study of the docetaxel/carboplatin combination versus docetaxel single-agent as second line treatment for patients with advanced/metastatic non-small cell lung cancer. BMC Cancer	Qi (2012)[126]
New Agent	
Herbst, 2010[136] Vandetanib plus docetaxel versus docetaxel as second-line treatment for patients with advanced non-small-cell lung cancer (ZODIAC): a double-blind, randomized, phase 3 trial. Lancet Oncol	Qi (2012)[126] Qi (2011)[125] Yang (2010)[127]
De Boer, 2011[137] Vandetanib plus pemetrexed for the second-line treatment of advanced non-small-cell lung cancer: a randomized, double-blind phase III trial. J Clin Oncol	Qi (2011)[125] Qi (2012)[124]
Natale, 2011[138] Phase III trial of vandetanib compared with erlotinib in patients with previously treated advanced non-small-cell lung cancer. J Clin Oncol	Qi (2011)[125]

* The systematic review by Mountzios and colleagues in this second line section did not overlap with any trials identified by our search or TEP, and is thus not included in this table

The remaining 15 trials were not found in any of the systematic reviews.[123, 139-153] Table S3 has the details of these trials. We discuss these here in the order in which they emerged into clinical practice: docetaxel, followed by pemetrexed, then tyrosine kinase inhibitors (TKI), and finally newer agents.

Docetaxel

We identified one new trial of docetaxel. Fossella and coleagues 373 patients were randomized to receive either docetaxel 100mg/m2, docetaxel 75mg/m2 versus a regimen of either vinorelbine or ifosfamide.[151] Overall survival was not significantly different between the three groups, 5.5 months for docetaxel 100mg/m2, 5.7 months for docetaxel 75mg/m2 and 5.6 months for vinorelbine/ifosfamide. However, the 1-year survival was significantly greater with docetaxel 75mg 32% (95% CI: 23-40) than with vinorelbine/ifosfamide 19% (12-26). The overall response rates for both of the docetaxel arms were significantly higher than that of the vinorelbine/ifosfamide arm with 10.8% for docetaxel 100mg/m2, 6.7% for docetaxel 75mg/m2 and 0.8% with vinorelbine/ifosfamide (p=.001 and p=.036, respectively).

Pemetrexed

Cullen et al, randomized 588 patients to either standard or high-dose pemetrexed.[145] The goal was to accrue 600 patients, however accrual was terminated after an interim analysis indicated a low probability of improved survival and numerically greater toxicity in the higher dose arm. Of the patients randomized, there was no statistically significant difference between the two groups in median survival reaching 6.7 months with the lower dose and 6.9 months with the higher dose (HR=1.0132, 95% CI: 0.837-1.226). Likewise there was no significant difference in overall response with 7.1% in the lower dose and 4.3% in the higher dose (P=0.1616).

TKI versus Cytotoxic Therapy

There were six trials comparing TKI to cytotoxic therapy.[139-144, 152] Ciuleanu et al, included 424 patients who were randomized to receive either erlotonib or chemotherapy.[139] About two-thirds of patients were positive for EGFR mutations. Median overall survival was 5.3 months (4.0-6.0) in the erlotinib group and 5.5 months (4.4-7.1) with chemotherapy (HR=0.96, 95% CI: 0.78-1.19; log-rank p=0.73). The response rate was also similar between the 2 groups with a RR of 7.9% (4.6-12.5) in the erlotinib group and 6.3% (3.5-10.4) in the chemotherapy group. The one-year survival was 26% (19-32) in the erlotinib group versus 24% (18-30) in the chemotherapy group.

Maruyama and colleagues randomized 489 patients to receive either gefitinib or docetaxel.[140] Patients were enrolled irrespective of EGFR receptor mutation status. There was no significant difference in overall survival, which was 11.5 months (95% CI: 9.8-14.0) in the gefitinib arm and 14.0 months (95% CI: 11.7-16.5)in the docetaxel arm (P=.330). However, for ORR gefitinib was statistically superior to docetaxel (22.5% v 12.8%, odds ratio, 2.14; 95% CI: 1.21-3.78; P=.009).

Sekine and colleagues assessed quality of life outcomes in the preceding study reported by Maruyama and colleagues.[142] This studied evaluated the quality of life differences between these two regimens and found gefitinib to have statistically significant benefits over docetaxel. The Functional Assessment of Cancer Therapy-Lung analysis was 23% for gefitinib versus 14% for docetaxel (P=0.023). The Trial Outcome Index was 21% vs 9% (P=0.002). There was no significant differences between treatments in Lung Cancer Subscale improvement rates (23% vs 20%, P=0.562). This study is the quality of life assessment outcome of a trial by Maruyama and colleagues, discussed above.[140]

Kim and colleagues randomized 1466 patients to either gefitinib or docetaxel.[141] Patients were enrolled irrespective of EGFR mutation status. Median overall survival was 7.6 months in the gefitinib group and 8.0 months in the docetaxel group. One-year survival was 32% for gefitinib and 34% for docetaxel.

Lee and colleagues randomized 161 patients to either gefitinib or docetaxel.[143] Patients were enrolled irrespective of EGFR mutation status. The overall survival was 14.1 months for gefitinib and 12.2 months for docetaxel (HR=0.870, 95% CI: 0.613-1.236, 2-sided p=0.4370). The objective response rate was statistically superior in the gefitinib group (28.1%) compared to the docetaxel group (7.6%) (P=0.0007).

Lastly, during peer review an abstract presented at the 2012 ASCO Annual Meeting was identified.[152] This study randomized 221 patients to erlotinib or docetaxel; all patients had wild type EGFR status. At a median follow-up of 20 months, progression-free survival favored treatment with docetaxel. Overall survival was not yet analyzed. We await full publication of these results, which will provide more complete analyses.

TKI As an Addition to Cytotoxic Therapy

This study of pemetrexed was added during peer review.[153] The study has been presented at the the 2011 ASCO Annual Meeting, but full publication is still pending. This was a phase II study in which 165 patients were randomized to receive either pemetrexed or pemetrexed plus erlotinib. The median progression-free survival was 2.9 months versus 3.2 months favoring combination therapy (HR=0.63, 95% CI 0.44-0.90). Overall survival also favored combination therapy (11.8

months vs. 7.8 months, HR=0.68, 95% CI 0.47-0.98). We await full publication of these results, which will provide more complete analyses, and confirmation in a phase III study.

TKI Plus Bevacizumab versus TKI Alone

Herbst and colleagues randomized 636 patients to either bevacizumab plus erlotinib or erlotinib alone.[144] Approximately 90 percent of patients had wild type EGFR receptor status. The overall survival did not differ between the two groups with the median overall survival of 9.3 months (IQR 4.1-21.6) in the bevacizumab arm compared to 9.2 months (IQR 3.8-20.2) in the erlotinib alone arm (HR=0.97, 95% CI: 0.80-1.18, p=0.7583). Objective response rate was much higher in the bevacizumab group (13% vs 6%).

Various Other Agents

There were seven trials of various other agents or doses.[123, 146-151, 153] Ready and colleagues randomized 106 patients to either the proapoptotic agent AT-101 or placebo in combination with docetaxel.[146] There was no significant difference in the median overall survival which was 7.8 months in the AT-101 arm and 5.9 months in the placebo arm (HR=0.82, 95% CI: 0.5-1.3, p=0.21). According to an independent review, the response rate and median PFS were not different between the arms, with the PFS for the AT-101 group of 7.5 weeks and 7.1 weeks for placebo (HR=1.04, p=0.57).

Ramlau and colleagues randomized 829 patients to either oral topotecan or IV docetaxel.[147] The median survival was higher with docetaxel at 30.7 weeks (95% CI: 28-34) compared to 27.9 weeks (95% CI: 24-31) with topotecan (p=.0568). Overall response rate was 5% (95% CI: 3-7%) for both docetaxel and topotecan. One-year survival was 29% (24-33%) for docetaxel and 25% (21-29%) for topotecan.

Paz-Ares and colleagues randomized 849 patients to either paclitaxel poliglumex or docetaxel.[148] The median survival was not different, at 6.9 months in each arm (HR 1.09, p=0.257). The 1-year survival was also similar with 25% in the paclitaxel poliglumex arm and 29% in the docetaxel arm (P=0.006).

Hermes and colleagues randomized 220 patients to either irinotecan plus carboplatin or etoposide plus carboplatin.[39, 154] Overall survival was better in the irinotecan group with a median survival of 8.5 months compared with 7.1 months in the etoposide group (etoposide relative to irinotecan HR=1.41; 95% CI: 1.06-1.87). The one-year survival rate was 34% for irinotecan and 24% for etoposide.

Krzakowski and colleagues randomized 551 patients to either vinflunine or docetaxel.[149] The median overall survival was 6.7 months (95% CI: 5.9-7.9) in the vinflunine group and 7.2 months (6.0-8.5) in the docetaxel group (HR=0.973, 95% CI: 0.805-1.176). The overall response rate was 4.4% for vinflunine and 5.5% for docetaxel treatment.

Finally, Schiller and colleagues randomized 150 patients to receive either pemetrexed alone, pemetrexed plus matuzumab 800mg/week, or pemetrexed plus matuzumab 1600mg/3 weeks.[150] There was a trend for improved OS in patients receiving matuzumab weekly compared to the every 3 weeks group with the former of 12.4 months and the latter 5.9 months. This was also greater than the 7.9 months of the pemetrexed group. Pooling the matuzumab arms gave an ORR of 11% compared to 5% for pemetrexed alone. Of note, all responses, except for one patient in the pemetrexed group, occurred in patients whose tumors expressed EGFR.

Table S3. Trials Not Included in Existing Systematic Reviews

Author; Date	N_{rand}	Comparison Agents/ N	Histology(%)**	EGFR mutation status (if relevant)	Median Survival, months (95% CI), p value	1-year survival % (95% CI), p value	Overall Response, % (95% CI), p value
Docetaxel							
Fossella, 2000[151]	373	D100mg/m2/125 D75mg/m2/125 V or I/123	A: 50 S: 27	NR	5.5 5.7 5.6	32(23-40) 19(12-26)	10.8 6.7, p=.001 0.8, p=.036
Pemetrexed							
Cullen, 2008[145]	588	Pem (standard dose)/295 Pem (hi dose)/293	NR	NR	6.7 6.9	NR	7.1 4.3, p=0.1616
TKI vs. Cytotoxic Therapy							
Ciuleanu, 2012[139]	424	E/203 Chemo/221	A: 50 S: 37	68% EGFR positive	5.3 (4.0-6.0) 5.5 (4.4-7.1) p=0.73	26 (19-32) 24 (18-30)	7.9(4.6-12.5) 6.3(3.5-10.4)
Maruyama, 2008[140]	489	Gf/245 D/244	A: 78 S: 16	Enrolled irrespective	11.5(9.8-14.0) 14.0(11.7-16.5) p=.330	NR	22.5 12.8, p=.009
Sekine, 2009[142]	490	Gf/245 D/244	Same as Maruyama, above		NR	NR	NR
Kim, 2008[141]	1466	Gf/733 D/733	A; 57 S; 25	57% EGFR mutation positive	7.6 8.0	NR	32 34
Lee, 2010[143]	161	Gf/82 D/79	A: 66 S: 21	Enrolled irrespective	14.1 12.2 p=0.4370	NR	28.1 7.6, p=0.0007
Garassino, 2012[152]	221	E/108 D/110	NR	100% EGFR wild-type	NR	NR	NR
TKI as an Addition to Cytotoxic Therapy							
Von Pawel, 2011[153]	165	Pem/83 Pem+E/76	Non-S: 100	NR	7.8 (5.3-10.4) 11.8 (8.2-16.7), P=0.019	NR	10.8 17.1
TKI Plus Bevacizumab vs. TKI Alone							
Herbst, 2011[144]	636	BE/319 E/317	A: 75 S: 4	90% EGFR wild type	9.3 9.2, p=0.7583	NR	13 6
Various							
Ready, 2011[146]	106	D+AT-101/53 DPl/52	A: 30 S: 56	NR	7.8 5.9, p=0.21	NR	NR
Ramlau, 2006[147]	829	T/414 D/415	A: 42 S: 41	NR	27.9weeks(24-31) 30.7weeks(28-34), p=.0568	25 (21-29) 29 (24-33)	5 5
Paz-Ares, 2008[148]	849	Px/427 D/422	NR	NR	6.9 6.9, p=0.257	25 29, p=0.006	NR
Krzakowski, 2010[149]	551	Vin/274 D/277	A; 43 S;35	NR	6.7(5.9-7.9) 7.2(6.0-8.5)	NR	4.4 5.5
Hermes, 2008[39]	220	Ir+Cb/105 Et+Cb/104	NR	NR	8.5 7.1 p=0.02	34 24	NR
Schiller, 2010[150]	150	Pem/50 PemMat (weekly)/51 PemMat (q3weeks)/49	A: 51 S: 31	EGFR expression status detectable (88%) vs. nondetectable (11%)	7.9 12.4 5.9	NR	5 11 (PemMat groups combined)

** A: Adenocarcinoma, S: squamous cell carcinoma

N_{rand}, number of patients randomized; NR, not reported; C, cisplatin; Cb, carboplatin; CI, confidence interval; D, docetaxel; Et, etoposide; G, gemcitabine; Ir, Irinotecan; P, paclitaxel; Vd, vindesine; MVP, mitomycin; Pem, pemetrexed; E, erlotinib; Gf, gefitinib; B, bevacizumab; Pl, placebo; BSC, best supportive care; T, topotecan; Ct, cetuximab; Vin, vinflunine; Mat, matuzumab; If, ifosfamide

Summary of Second-line therapy Trials Not in Existing Systematic Reviews

The summary of these trials not included in existing systematic reviews is:

- Considering data from first line and maintenance therapy studies in addition to second line studies, there are sufficient data to support the conclusion that histology type influences the effectiveness of potential treatments. Pemetrexed is more effective in nonsquamous NSCLC, while docetaxel is more effective in squamous NSCLC (GRADE=moderate).
- Tyrosine kinase inhibitors, when used as second-line therapy in patients unselected for EGFR mutation status, produce overall survival similar to docetaxel (GRADE=strong).
- There is insufficient data to support effectiveness of other drugs, or drugs in combinations, in second-line therapy (GRADE=moderate).
- The above second line studies are typically undertaken after evidence of disease progression, and should be distinguished from mainenance therapy, which is undertaken when a patient has at least stable disease during treatment (typically four cycles).

Toxicity of Second Line or Maintenance Agents

Analogous to the presentation in first line threatment, we present here a summary of Grade 3 or 4 toxicities from selected trials of second line agents, some of which are also used in maintenance therapy. As noted before, comparisons across trials should be avoided, and "numbers are provided only to give a general sense of the toxicity of the regimens."[2]

TABLE S4. Summary of Grade 3 or 4 Chemotherapy Toxicity (% Patients) from Large, Selected Trials of Maintenance or Second-line therapy

Regimen Dose (mg/m^2) and Administration Schedule [Reference]	Skin Rash	Diarrhea	Infection/ Infestation	Hypertension	Fatigue	Bleeding	Nausea	Febrile Neutropenia	Neutropenia
Erlotinib 150 mg/day [Cappuzzo 2010[155]]	9	2	1	NR	NR	NR	NR	NR	NR
Erlotinib 110 mg/daily [Ciuleanu 2012[139]]	5	18	NR	NR	3	NR	5	NR	NR
Bevacizumab 15 mg/kg; erlotinib 150 mg/daily [Herbst 2011[144]]	NR	NR	NR	15	NR	3	NR	NR	NR
Pemetrexed 500 mg/m^2 [Cullen 2008[145]]	0.3	1.4	2.4	NR	3.1	NR	1.4	1.4	2.1

Abbreviations: AUC = area under curve; hr = hour; mg=milligrams; m^2= meters squared; min = minutes; NR = not reported; NSCLC = non-small cell lung cancer.

KEY QUESTION 3. For patients with metastatic NSCLC what is the benefit of maintenance therapy following first line chemotherapy regimens compared with no maintenance therapy?

We identified three systematic reviews of maintenance therapy published since 2010.[3, 20, 156] Details of these systematic reviews are in Table M1. The most comprehensive and best quality review was completed by Zhang and colleague.[3] It met 10 of the 11 AMSTAR criteria and identified eight trials with a total of 3,736 patients with nonprogressing NSCLC. Trials were of either a continuous or switch strategy and were compared to either placebo or observation. Of the nine trials, three employed a continuous maintenance strategy[157-159] while six utilized a switch strategy.[155, 159, 160, 161-164]

Treatment of Metastatic Non-Small Cell Lung Cancer

Table M1. Maintenance Systematic Reviews Published Since 2010

Author (Year)	Search End Date	What was compared	Trials included; Total Number of Patients First Author, Year Title. Journal*	Outcomes Reported				Conclusions per abstract:
				Overall Survival	Progression Free Survival	Overall Response Rate	Adverse Events / Other Outcomes Reported	
Zhang et al. (2011)[3]	Aug 2010	Erlotinib vs. Gefitinib vs. Placebo; Gemcitabine vs. BSC or observation; pemetrexed vs. placebo and BSC; Bevacizumab and erlotinib vs. bevacizumab and placebo; erlotinib vs. observation	8 trials; 3,736 pts Capuzzo, 2010 Perol, 2010 Ciuleanu, 2009 Brodowicz, 2006 Belani, 2010 Fidias, 2009 Miller, 2009 Kabbinavar, 2010 Surmont, 2010	X	X		X (Adverse Events)	Maintenance therapy with either a continuous or a switch strategy significantly increases OS and PFS compared with placebo or observation. However, the benefits must be balanced against toxicity.
Qi et al. (2012)[156a]	March 2011	Pemetrexed or Erlotinib vs. Placebo	5 trials; 3,634 pts Capuzzo, 2010 Herbst, 2005 Perol, 2010 Ciuleanu, 2009 Paz-Ares, 2011	X	X			Maintenance therapy with either erlotinib or pemetrexed has clinically and statistically significant advantage over placebo observation.
Mountzios et al. (2011)[20b]	Feb 2010	SATURN: Erlotinib vs. Placebo; ATLAS: erlotinib + bevacizumab vs. bevacizumab	2 trials; 1,768 pts Capuzzo, 2009 Miller, 2009	X	X	X	X (Adverse Events); Risk of death	Based on the results of the SATURN and ATLAS studies, the use of erlotinib as maintenance therapy is becoming a treatment option for patients with good performance status who respond to first-line chemotherapy.

*Full trial references are listed below
Reviews are listed in order of comprehensiveness (total patients, included trials)
[a] Qi contains two trials (Capuzzo 2010 and Ciuleanu 2009), totaling 1,552 patients, that are included in Zhang 2011.
[b] Mountzios contains two maintenance trials (Capuzzo 2010 and Miller 2009), totaling 1,768 patients, that are included in Zhang 2011.

Trial References, by Systematic Review, for Table M1.

Zhang et al. (2011):

- **Pérol** M, Zalcman G, Monnet I, et al. Final results from the IFCT-GFPC 0502 phase III study: maintenance therapy in advanced NSCLC with either gemcitabine (G) or erlotinib (E) versus observation (O) after cisplatin-gemcitabine induction chemotherapy (CT), with predefined second-line treatment [abstract]. Ann Oncol. 2010; 21 (suppl 8): viii 124.

- **Cappuzzo** F, Ciuleanu T, Stelmakh L, et al; SATURN investigators. Erlotinib as maintenance treatment in advanced non-small-cell lung cancer: a multicentre, randomised, placebo controlled phase 3 study. Lancet Oncol. 2010; 11 (6): 521 - 529.

- **Ciuleanu** T, Brodowicz T, Zielinski C, et al. Maintenance pemetrexed plus best supportive care versus placebo plus best supportive care for non-small-cell lung cancer: a randomised, double-blind, phase 3 study. Lancet. 2009; 374(9699): 1432- 1440.

- **Miller** VA, Das A, Rossi M. A randomized, double-blind, placebo-controlled, phase IIIb trial (ATLAS) comparing bevacizumab (B) therapy with or without erlotinib (E) after completion of chemotherapy with B for first-line treatment of locally advanced, recurrent, or metastatic non-small cell lung cancer (NSCLC) [abstract LBA8002]. J Clin Oncol. 2009; 27 (suppl 1): 18S.

- **Kabbinavar** FF, Miller VA, Johnson BE, et al. Overall survival (OS) in ATLAS, a phase IIIb trial comparing bevacizumab (B) therapy with or without erlotinib (E) after completion of chemotherapy (chemo) with B for first-line treatment of locally advanced, recurrent, or metastatic non-small cell lung cancer (NSCLC) [abstract 7526]. J Clin Oncol. 2010; 28 (suppl): 15S.

- **Brodowicz** T, Krzakowski M, Zwitter M, et al; Central European Cooperative Oncology Group CECOG. Cisplatin and gemcitabine first-line chemotherapy followed by maintenance gemcitabine or best supportive care in advanced nonsmall cell lung cancer: a phase III trial. Lung Cancer. 2006; 52 (2): 155 - 163.

Treatment of Metastatic Non-Small Cell Lung Cancer

- **Belani** CP, Waterhouse DM, Ghazal H, et al. Phase III study of maintenance gemcitabine (G) and best supportive care (BSC) versus BSC, following standard combination therapy with gemcitabine-carboplatin (G-Cb) for patients with advanced non-small cell lung cancer (NSCLC) [abstract 7506]. J Clin Oncol. 2010; 28 (suppl): 15S.
- **Fidias** PM, Dakhil SR, Lyss AP, et al. Phase III study of immediate compared with delayed docetaxel after front-line therapy with gemcitabine plus carboplatin in advanced non small-cell lung cancer. J Clin Oncol. 2009; 27 (4): 591 - 598.
- **Surmont** VF, Gaafar RM, Scagliotti GV, et al. A double-blind, randomized, placebo-controlled phase III intergroup study of gefitinib (G) in patients (pts) with advanced NSCLC, non-progressing after first-line platinum-based chemotherapy (EORTC 08021-ILCP 01/03) [abstract]. Ann Oncol. 2010; 21 (suppl 8): viii 124.

Qi et al. (2012)

- **Cappuzzo** F, Ciuleanu T, Stelmakh L, et al. Erlotinib as maintenance treatment in advanced non-small-cell lung cancer: a multi-centre, randomized, placebo-controlled phase 3 study. Lancet Oncol 2010; 11: 521-9.
- **Herbst** RS, Prager D, Hermann R, et al. TRIBUTE: a phase III trial of erlotinib hydrochloride (OSI-774) combined with carboplatin and paclitaxel chemotherapy in advanced non-small-cell lung cancer. J Clin Oncol 2005; 23: 5892-9.
- **Ciuleanu** T, Brodowicz T, Zielinski C, et al. Maintenance pemetrexed plus best supportive care versus placebo plus best supportive care for non-small-cell lung cancer: a randomized, double-blind, phase 3 study. Lancet 2009;374:1432-40
- **Perol** M, Chouaid C, Milleron BJ, et al. Maintenance with either gemcitabine or erlotinib versus observation with predefined second-line treatment after cisplatin–gemcitabine induction chemotherapy in advanced NSCLC: IFCT-GFPC 0502 phase III study. J Clin Oncol 2010;28(Suppl):15s (abstr 7507)
- **Paz-Ares** LG, De Marinis F, Dediu M, et al. PARAMOUNT: Phase III study of maintenance pemetrexed (pem) plus best supportive care (BSC) versus placebo plus BSC immediately following induction treatment with pem plus cisplatin for advanced nonsquamous non-small cell lung cancer (NSCLC). J Clin Oncol 2011;29(Suppl):18s (abstr CRA7510)

Mountzios et al. (2011)

- **Cappuzzo** F, Coudert B, Wierzbicki R, et al. Efficacy and safety of erlotinib as first-line maintenance in NSCLC following non-progression with chemotherapy: results from the phase III SATURN study [abstract no. A2.1]. 13th World Conference on Lung Cancer IASCL 2009; 2009 Jul 31- Aug 4; San Francisco (CA).
- **Miller** V, O'Connor P, Soh CH, et al. A randomized, double blind, placebo controlled, phase IIIb trial (ATLAS) comparing bevacizumab therapy with or without erlotinib, after completion of chemotherapy with bevacizumab for 1st-line treatment of locally-advanced, recurrent, or metastatic non-small cell lung cancer (NSCLC) [abstract no. LBA8002]. J Clin Oncol 2009; 27: 18s.

In the trials examining continuous maintenance therapy, there was a trend towards benefits in the overall survival, however this did not quite reach statistical significance (HR=0.88; 95% CI: 0.74-1.04; p=.15). There was no evidence of heterogeneity between the studies (p=.66, I2=0%). The first of these trials accrued 215 patients and continued patients on gemcitabine after an initial therapy of gemcitabine and cisplatin. Overall survival was 10.2 months in the maintenance group compared to 8.1 months in the best supportive care group (HR=0.79; 95% CI: 0.57-1.11).[157] Another trial of 255 patients on gemcitabine following gemcitabine and cisplatin found overall survival to be 8 months in the maintenance group versus 9.3 months in the best supportive care group (HR=0.97; 95% CI: 0.72-1.30).[158] The last of these trials accrued 309 patients, treating them with gemcitabine after gemcitabine and cisplatin and favored continued maintenance, though specific data were not reported.[159]

The six trials examining switch maintenance therapy found a clinically and statistically significant 15% improvement in OS when compared to the placebo or observation groups (HR=0.85; 95% CI: 0.79-0.92; p<.001). There was no evidence of heterogeneity (p=.77, I2=0%). There were two trials of cytotoxic agents. The first trial accrued 309 patients and treated patients with docetaxel after gemcitabine and carboplatin. The overall survival of the maintenance therapy group was 12.3 months compared to 9.7 months in the best supportive care group (HR=0.81, 95% CI: 0.63-1.03).[165] The other trial included 663 patients treated with pemetrexed after platinum-doublet chemotherapy versus placebo and found overall survival to be 13.4 and 10.6 months (HR=0.79, 95% CI: 0.65-0.95).[164] There were four trials of molecular-targeted agents. Two trials were combined to give 768 patients treated with bevacizumab and either erlotinib or placebo after bevacizumab and platinum-doublet chemotherapy. The erlotinib group had an overall survival of 15.9 months versus 13.9 in the placebo group (HR=0.90, 95% CI: 0.74-1.09; p=0.2686).[161, 162] A trial of 889 patients receiving erlotinib or placebo after platinum-doublet chemotherapy found the overall survival to be 12 in the erlotinib group and 11 in the placebo group.[155] Another study of erlotinib included 310 patients and compared it to observation following gemcitabine and cisplatin. The overall survival hazard ratio was 0.91 (95% CI: 0.80-1.04) in favor of the maintenance therapy.[159] The last of these studies included 173 patients treated with gefitinib or placebo after platinum-doublet chemotherapy and found an overall survival of 10.9 months in the treatment arm versus 9.4 months (HR=0.87, 95% CI: 0.80-0.95).[163]

Overall, these nine trials comprised 3,736 patients. When comparing continuous and switch maintenance therapies, the interaction test found no statistically significant difference in overall survival (HR=0.88 vs. 0.85; interaction p=0.78). This result was interpreted as meaning that there is no evidence to conclude superiority for either the continuous or the switch approach. Within the trials of switch maintenance, a subgroup analysis revealed that there was no statistically significant difference in overall survival between the cytotoxic and tyrosine kinase inhibitor agents. Again, the conclusion is that there is no evidence to support that one approach is superior to the other.

The other two systematic reviews were more targeted. The first review identified 5 trial including 3,634 patients.[156] Three of these trials were of erlotinib versus either placebo or gemcitabine. Two of the trials were of pemetrexed versus placebo. Two of the trials were included in the review by Zhang.[155, 166] Both regimens led to significant improvement in overall survival compared with placebo or observation (erlotinib HR=0.90, 95% CI: 0.83-0.98; pemetrexed HR=0.79; 95% CI:

0.65-0.95) and relative hazards ratio showed no significant difference between the two agents (HR=0.88; 95% CI: 0.71-1.08, p=0.22). These results are compatible with the conclusions of the review by Zhang and colleagues. However, pemetrexed was superior to erlotinib in the outcome of progression free survival. The other systematic review included the SATURN and ATLAS trials which studied erlotinib versus placebo and erlotinib and bevacizumab versus bevacizumab alone.[20] There were 2 trials including 1768 patients. In the SATURN trial, patients in the erlotinib arm had a better response rate (12% vs 5%), PFS (12 vs. 11.1 weeks; HR=0.71; 95% CI: 0.62,0.82; p<0.0001) and better overall survival (12 vs. 11 months, HR=0.81, 95% CI: 0.70, 0.95; p=0.0088). The ATLAS trial found an improvement in progression free survival of 4.76 versus 3.75 months (HR=0.722; 95% CI: 0.592, 0.881; p<0.0012).

Finally, we identified four additional trials.[167-171] Details of these trials are presented in Table M2. The first was a quality of life assessment of the study by Ciuleanu, included in the systematic review by Zhang.[168] This trial treated 663 patients with pemetrexed or placebo after platinum-based therapy. The primary outcome was time to worsening of symptoms and this was longer in the pemetrexed group for pain (HR=0.76, 95% CI: 0.59-0.99; p=0.041) and hemoptysis (HR=0.58, 95% CI: 0.34-0.97; p=0.038). The PARAMOUNT trial of pemetrexed versus placebo treated 539 patients who had undergone therapy with pemetrexed and cisplatin.[167] Within the 359 patients treated with pemetrexed, there was a significant reduction in the risk of disease progression compared to the placebo group (HR=0.62, 95% CI: 0.49-0.79; p<0.0001). In addition, the median progression free survival in the pemetrexed group was 4.1 months (95% CI: 3.2-4.6) versus 2.8 months (95% CI: 2.6-3.1) in the placebo group. The results of the PARAMOUNT trial were recently updated in abstract form at the 2012 ASCO Annual Meeting.[171] Continuation maintenance therapy with pemetrexed resulted in a 22 percent reduction in the risk of death at a median follow-up of 12.5 months. The INFORM trial by Zhang and colleagues randomized Chinese patients with advanced NCSLC who had received four cycles of platinum-based doublet therapy to gefitinib pr placebo.[170] Progression-free survival was approximately doubled from 2.6 to 4.8 months; there was no difference in overall survival. Adverse events, primarily rash, diarrhea, and liver function abnormalities, were much more common in patients taking gefitinib. Lastly, there was a trial of thalidomide versus placebo in 722 patients who had been treated with gemcitabine and carboplatin.[169] Thalidomide did not improve overall survival as the median duration in the placebo group was 8.9 months compared to 8.5 months in the thalidomide arm (HR=1.13, 95% CI: 0.97-1.32; p=.12). Unfortunately, the risk of thrombotic stroke was increased by 74% in the thalidomide group (HR=1.74, 95% CI: 1.20-2.52; p=.003). In addition survival was significantly worse in those patients who had nonsquamous histology. In summary, two of these trials reported benefits in additional outcomes for maintenance therapy with pemetrexed compared to placebo, while two other trials did not support any beneficial clinical effect for maintenance treatment with paclitaxel or thalidomide.

Treatment of Metastatic Non-Small Cell Lung Cancer

Table M2. Trials Not Included in Existing Systematic Reviews

Author; Date	Study or Setting	Maintenance following	Treatments being compared	Outcomes	Conclusions per abstract:
Belani et al.; 2012[168]	QOL assessment of study by Ciuleanu (Lancet 2009) included in Zhang (2011)	Four cycles of platinum-based induction therapy	Best supportive care plus placebo or pemetrexed (500 mg/m² every 21 days)	QOL (Lung Cancer Symptom Scale)	Longer time to worsening was recorded for pain (hazard ratio [HR] 0.76, 95% CI: 0.59-0.99; p = 0.041) and haemoptysis (HR=0.58, 95% CI: 0.34-0.97, p = 0.038) with pemetrexed than with placebo; no other significant differences in analyses of time to worsening were noted. Additional longitudinal analyses showed a greater increase in loss of appetite in the pemetrexed group than in the placebo group (4.3 mm vs. 0.2 mm; p=0.028). Quality of life during maintenance therapy with pemetrexed is similar to placebo, except for a small increase in loss of appetite, and significantly delayed worsening of pain and haemoptysis. In view of the improvements in overall and progression-free survival noted with pemetrexed maintenance therapy, such treatment is an option for patients with advanced non-squamous NSCLC who have not progressed after platinum-based induction therapy.
Paz-Ares et al.; 2012[167]	PARAMOUNT trial; multicenter phase III	Induction therapy with pemetrexed plus cisplatin	Best supportive care plus either placebo or maintenance with pemetrexed (500 mg/m² every 21 days)	Progression-free survival; adverse events	Among the 359 patients randomized to continuation maintenance with pemetrexed, there was a significant reduction in the risk of disease progression over the placebo group (HR=0.62, 95% CI: 0.49-0.79, p<0.0001). The median progression-free survival, measured from randomization, was 4.1 months (95% CI: 3.2-4.6) for pemetrexed and 2.8 months (2.6-3.1) for placebo. Continuation maintenance with pemetrexed is an effective and well tolerated treatment option for patients with advanced non-squamous NSCLC with good performance status who have not progressed after induction therapy with pemetrexed plus cisplatin.
Paz-Ares et al.; 2012[171]				Overall survival	Continuation maintenance therapy with pemetrexed resulted in a 22 percent reduction in the risk of death at a median follow-up of 12.5 months.
Zhang et al.; 2012[170]	INFORM trial; multicenter phase III trial in China	Four cycles of platinum-based doublet therapy	Gefitinib (250 mg/day) or placebo	Overall survival, progression-free survival, adverse events	Progression-free survival was significantly longer with gefitinib (n=148) than placebo (n=148) (median progression-free survival of 4.8 months [95% CI: 3.2-8.5] vs. 2.6 months [95% CI: 1.6-2.8]; hazard ratio [HR]: 0.42, 95%CI: 0.33-0.55, p<0.0001). Adverse events occurred more frequently with gefitinib treatment.
Lee et al.; 2009[169]	Multicenter phase III	Gemcitabine and carboplatin every 3 weeks for 4 cycles	Thalidomide or placebo capsules (100-200 mg/daily) beginning at the start of chemotherapy and continuing for up to 2 years.	Overall survival, progression-free survival, response rate, grade 3/4 toxicity, and quality of life	The median OS rates were 8.9 months (placebo) and 8.5 months (thalidomide). The hazard ratio (HR) was 1.13 (95% CI: 0.97-1.32; P=.12). The 2-year survival rate was 16% and 12% in the placebo and thalidomide arms, respectively. The risk of having a thrombotic event was increased by 74% in the thalidomide group: HR of 1.74 (95% CI: 1.20-2.52; P=0.003). In this large trial of patients with NSCLC, thalidomide in combination with chemotherapy did not improve survival overall, but increased the risk of thrombotic events. Unexpectedly, survival was significantly worse in patients with nonsquamous history.

Summary of Key Question 3: Maintenance Therapy

- Maintenance therapy improves overall survival (GRADE=High).
- Maintenance therapy with gefitinib significantly prolonged preogression-free survival compared with placebo in patients from east Asia with advanced NSCLC who achieved disease control after first-line chemotherapy (GRADE=high).
- There is insufficient evidence to reach conclusions regarding whether a continuous or a switch strategy is superior (GRADE=Very low). However, two drugs have been approved for switch therapy.
- Differences in survival in placebo-controlled trials of erlotinib or cytotoxic agents are sufficiently small that head-to-head comparisons will be required before strong conclusions can be reached about comparative effectiveness.

KEY QUESTION 4. What is the relative cost and cost-effectiveness of the different approaches in Key Questions 1-3?

Our literature review identified one systematic review of cost-effectiveness analyses and 21 cost-effectiveness analyses published since 2010. Of the latter, eight analyses concerned first-line therapy, seven analyses concerned second-line therapy, six analyses concerned maintenance therapy, and one concerned third line therapy. A single publication could deal with more than one kind of therapy. Eleven analyses assessed erlotinib, nine analyses assessed pemetrexed, five analyses assessed bevacizumab, five analyses assessed docetaxel, and a number of other agents were assessed less frequently (analyses could assess more than one agent). Four studies assessed cost-effectiveness from a US payor perspective, while the remainder used non-US payor perspectives. Almost all studies used life expectancy or quality-adjusted life years (QALYs) as the measure of outcome. Details about the 22 analyses are presented in Table CE1.

The systematic review by Bongers and colleagues was published in 2012 and searched PubMed, EMBASE, and the Health Economic Evaluations database from 2001 through October 2010. The authors identified 6 prior systematic reviews, six cost-effectiveness analyses, and 6 cost-utility analyses. Four assessments of first-line therapy were included, as were 6 assessments of second-line therapy. The authors noted numerous methodological weaknesses in the included studies. Their overall conclusions were:

- Due to the small number of studies, heterogeneity between studies and lack of a clear and consistent definition of best supportive care in each study, strong conclusions cannot be drawn
- The estimates of key parameters, model assumptions, and calculations in modeling studies were often poorly reported.
- However, there was reasonable consensus between studies that gemcitabine-cisplatin is a cost-effective option for first-line treatment of non-small cell lung cancer, although pemetrexed-cisplatin appears more effective for non-squamous-cell carcinoma
- In second line treatment, docetaxel appears to be cost-effective compared with best supportive care, while erlotinib may be a cost-effective alternative compared to docetaxel.

Treatment of Metastatic Non-Small Cell Lung Cancer

Table CE1. Cost-Effectiveness Analyses Published Since 2010

Author (Year)	Which treatments are assessed?	Where are the data from?	Perspective of the analysis*	QALYs	Life expectancy	Other	Conclusions per abstract:
First-Line Therapy							
Wu et al. (2011)	rh-endostatin	Single study: J Clin Oncol 2005; 23 (suppl): Abstract 7138	Non-US payer		X		The addition of rh-endostatin to standard first-line chemotherapy is unlikely to be cost-effective
Goulart and Ramsey (2011)	Bevacizumab	Single study: ECOG4599	US payer	X			Bevacizumab does not appear to be cost-effective when added to chemotherapy in patients with advanced NSCLC
Ahn et al. (2011)	Bevacizumab	Multiple studies	Non-US payer	X	X		BevCG (bevacizumab + cisplatin + gemcitabine) is more costly but associated with additional life years in Korea and Taiwan
Joerger et al. (2011)	Cetuximab	Single study: FLEX	Non-US payer	X			The addition of cetuximab to standard first-line chemotherapy in patients with epidermal growth factor receptor-expressing advanced NSCLC cannot be recommended to date, due to a high Incremental Cost-Effectiveness Ratio compared with other health care interventions
Stanisic et al. (2010)	Bevacizumab	Multiple studies	Societal perspective is France, Germany, Italy, Spain			Progression free survival	Bevacizumab-based treatment can result in substantial cost savings in progression-free patients with metastatic NSCLC
Bischoff et al. (2010)	Bevacizumab, pemetrexed	Multiple studies	Non-US payer		X		Clinical benefits with bevacizumab plus cisplatin and gemcitabine therapy are achieved at a lower monthly cost than pemetrexed plus gemcitabine doublet therapy
Giuliani et al. (2010)	Bevacizumab, pemetrexed	Multiple studies	Non-US payer		X		Bevacizumab-based therapy can be considered as a cost-effective option when compared to chemotherapy treatments such as pemetrexed for the treatment of advanced NSCLC
Thongprasert et al. (2011)	Carboplatin and paclitaxel	Single study: Chang Mai Hospital	Non-US payer	X			Carboplatin plus paclitaxel are not cost-effective at a threshold of 100,000 Baht (Thailand)
Second-line therapy							
Bradbury et al. (2010)	Erlotinib	BR.21 trial database, Canada	Non-US payer			Incremental cost-effectiveness ratio (2007 Canadian dollars to life-years gained)	With an incremental cost-effectiveness ratio of $94,638 per life-year gained, erlotinib treatment for patients with previously treated advanced non–small cell lung cancer is marginally cost-effective. The use of molecular predictors of benefit for targeted agents may help identify more or less cost-effective subgroups for treatment.
Asukai et al. (2010)	Pemetrexed, docetaxel		Non-US payer; Spain				Pemetrexed as a second-line treatment option for patients with a predominantly non-squamous histology in NSCLC is a cost-effective alternative to docetaxel according to the € 30000/QALY threshold commonly accepted in Spain.
Thongprasert et al. (2012)	Docetaxel, pemetrexed, erlotinib, gefitinib	Single study: INTEREST	Non-US payer	X			Gefitinib is a dominant cost-saving strategy compared with docetaxel

Treatment of Metastatic Non-Small Cell Lung Cancer

Author (Year)	Which treatments are assessed?	Where are the data from?	Perspective of the analysis*	QUALYs	Life expectancy	Other	Conclusions per abstract:
Cromwell et al. (2011)	Erlotinib, docetaxel	Single study: Own institution data	Non-US payer Payor perspective is Canadian provincial health care system		X		Erlotinib and docetaxel are statistically equivalent in terms of treatment cost and overall survival
Horgan et al. (2011)	Docetaxel, gefitinib Third line therapy is assessed	Single study: INTEREST	Non-US payer Canada cost perspective	X		Adverse events	The modest increase in cost associated with gefitinib supports its use as an alternative to docetaxel as second-line treatment of advanced NSCLC particularly given the improvements in QoL, patient preference for oral therapy and better toxicity profile with gefitinib
Vergnenegre et al. (2011)	Docetaxel, pemetrexed	Single study: GFPC 05-06	Non-US payer	X		Adverse events	Second line treatment for NSCLC is more cost-effective with docetaxel than with pemetrexed
Lewis et al. (2010)	Erlotinib, docetaxel	Multiple studies	Non-US payer From perspective of UK NHS, probably relevant to VA	X			In general, erlotinib appeared to generate similar overall survival, an increase in QALYs and a small reduction in NHS costs compared with docetaxel, due to lower adverse event and drug administration costs

Maintenance Therapy

Author (Year)	Which treatments are assessed?	Where are the data from?	Perspective of the analysis*	QUALYs	Life expectancy	Other	Conclusions per abstract:
Vergnenegre et al. (2012)	Erlotinib	Single study: SATURN	Non-US payer		X		Erlotinib is a cost-effective treatment option when used as first line maintenance therapy
Matter-Walstra et al. (2012)	Pemetrexed	Multiple studies	Non-US payer Payor perspective is Swiss Health Care System	X			Switch maintenance with pemetrexed inpatients with advanced nonsquamous-cell lung cancer is not cost-effective
Nuijten et al. (2011)	Erlotinib, pemetrexed	Multiple studies	Non-US payer		X	Adverse events	Erlotinib appears to be a cost-saving treatment alternative to pemetrexed, producing comparable survival benefits, based on indirect comparison at a lower cost
Banz et al. (2011)	Erlotinib, pemetrexed	Multiple studies	Non-US payer			Adverse events	Erlotinib maintenance therapy in patients with advanced NSCLC causes lower AE management costs then pemetrexed maintenance therapy
Carlson et al. (2011)	Erlotinib	Single study: Own institution	US payer			Costs	The overall budget impact to a health plan of expanding the use of erlotinib from the 2nd/3rd line advanced NSCLC setting to maintenance setting was relatively small
Klein et al. (2010)	Pemetrexed, bevacizumab, erlotinib About nonsquamous NSCLC	Multiple studies	US payer		X		Compared with observation and other agents used and/or reimbursed for maintenance therapy in advanced NSCLC, pemetrexed may be considered cost-effective, particularly in patients with nonsquamous cell histology

Other Therapy

Author (Year)	Which treatments are assessed?	Where are the data from?	Perspective of the analysis*	QUALYs	Life expectancy	Other	Conclusions per abstract:
Cromwell et al. (2012)	Erlotinib Third line therapy is assessed	Single study: Local Data	Non-US payer		X	X	Erlotinib may be an effective and cost-effective third-line treatment for advanced NSCLC compared to best supportive care

Our review identified 22 cost-effectiveness analyses published since 2010, of which four overlapped with the systematic review by Bongers and colleagues. We obtained additional information from our TEP to focus our assessment on the following key sub-questions:

First-line Therapy

- Which platinum-doublet is the most cost-effective therapy in squamous and in non-squamous histology types?
- In non-squamous NSCLC, is the carboplatin-paclitaxel-bevacizumab option more cost-effective than platinum-pemetrexed?

Second-line Therapy

- Which of the three approved agents (docetaxel, pemetrexed for non-squamous histology, or erlotinib) is more cost-effective?

Maintenance Therapy

- Which approach is more cost-effective: switch maintenance with pemetrexed, continuation maintenance therapy with pemetrexed or erlotinib?

Key Sub-question 4.1. Which platinum-doublet is the most cost-effective therapy in squamous and in non-squamous histology types?

The review by Bongers and colleagues concluded that there was a "reasonable consensus" that gemcitabine + cisplatin was more cost-effective than other doublet options assessed.[172] In the three studies used to reach this conclusion, the comparison options were paclitaxel-cisplatin, gemcitabine-paclitaxel, docetaxel-cisplatinum, vinorelbine-cisplatin, and pemetrexed-cisplatin. The payer perspectives were the Dutch health insurance system, the UK health care system, and a US payer. The study assessing pemetrexed (discussed in more detail, below) concluded that pemetrexed-cisplatin is more cost-effective than cisplatin-gemcitabine for patients with non-squamous disease.

Our search identified eight cost-effectiveness analyses of first-line therapy, but two dealt with agents that were not of interest (rh endostatin[173] and cetuximab[174]) and five dealt with bevacizumab (discussed below). Of the remaining two, one assessed the cost-effectiveness of cisplatin + etoposide compared to carboplatin + paclitaxel, using data from a single Thai hospital,[175] and was judged by our TEP to be not of interest for this review. Thus, there are no new cost-effectiveness analyses since the review by Bongers and colleagues that are relevant to this key sub-question. However, Key Question 1 for this review, about first-line therapy, identified one high quality systematic review by the CCO that concluded that "a combination of a platinum agent plus a new agent continues to be the standard of care" and "as differences between regimens are small, toxicity and patient preference should help guide regiment choice."[2] However, the CCO does note the meta-analysis by Le Chevalier that reported a trend toward improved survival with gemcitabine combinations. Eight clinical trials published since that review was completed in aggregate reach the same conclusion – no particular combination has been shown to be consistently superior in terms of effectiveness outcomes. In the absence of clinically important differences in effectiveness, then differences in the costs of the agents, and possibly the cost of treating different treatment toxicities, will drive any differences in cost-effectiveness. An addendum to the CCO review, restricted to pemetrexed, concluded that "data are compelling to recommend that pemetrexed should not be used in the treatment of squamous cell carcinomas for first line treatment" and "on the other hand, these data are not sufficiently compelling to recommend that pemetrexed be used preferentially over all other new agents in doublet therapy to treat adenocarcinoma in first line settings."

Key Sub-question 4.2. In non-squamous NSCLC, is the carboplatin-paclitaxel-bevacizumab option more cost-effective than platinum-pemetrexed?

This combination was not assessed in the review by Bongers and colleagues, but the cost-effectiveness of bevacizumab was the subject of five recent cost-effectiveness analyses, although none were of exactly this comparison. Four of these analyses were supported by the maker of bevacizumab.[176, 177, 178, 179] All three concluded that bevacizumab was a cost-effective approach to care in the following situations: bevacizumab + cisplatin + gemcitabine compared to pemetrexed + cisplatin in non-squamous cell histology, using an Italian payer perspective;[178] bevacizumab + cisplatin + gemcitabine compared to cisplatin + pemetrexed in non-squamous cell histology, using a Korean and Taiwanese health payer perspective;[176] the same combination using the payer perspective of Italy and Germany;[179] and an analysis that combined together the results of two trials, which compared the addition of bevacizumab to either cisplatin + gemcitabine or carboplatin + paclitaxel, and used a societal perspective including time off from work in France, Germany, Italy and Spain.[177]

The one non-industry funded analysis used a US payer perspective and compared the addition of bevacizumab to carboplatin + paclitaxel versus carboplatin + paclitaxel alone.[180] Data about outcomes came from the ECOG 4599 trial. Costs came from Medicare data. The discount rate for future costs and QALYs was 3% per year. The main result was the incremental cost-effectiveness ratio (ICER). Numerous sensitivity analyses were performed. The principal result was that the ICER was $560,000 per QALY gained, or $309,000 per life-year gained, for the addition of bevacizumab to the carboplatin + paclitaxel treatment. The results were most sensitive to the time for survival without progression while on treatment and the number of bevacizumab cycles. In order to reach a value of $100,000 per QALY gained, the addition of bevacizumab would have to result in a mean overall survival advantage of 1.3 years (while holding other model parameters constant). Alternatively, in order to reach the same $100,000/QALY threshold, the acquisition cost of bevacizumab would have to drop to $885, all other model parameters being held constant. The overall conclusion of the authors was that "bevacizumab does not appear to be cost-effective when added to chemotherapy in patients with advanced NSCLC, based on approximate cost-effectiveness thresholds that have been identified in the United States."

Key Sub-question 4.3 Which of the three approved agents (docetaxel, pemetrexed for non-squamous histology, or erlotinib) is more cost-effective?

The review by Bongers and colleagues concluded that "docetaxel appears to be cost-effective compared to best supportive care, while erlotinib may be a cost-effective alternative compared with docetaxel."[172] These conclusions were based on the results of 6 cost-effectiveness analyses, 3 of them published in 2010 and this also included in our assessment.[181-183] The other 3 analyses assessed the cost-effectiveness of docetaxel, in two of these docetaxel was compared to best supportive care and in one compared to pemetrexed and erlotinib. The two cost-effectiveness analyses comparing docetaxel with best supportive care both concluded that second line treatment with docetaxel had an incremental cost-effectiveness ratio well under conventional US thresholds for considering a treatment to be cost-effective: about $32,000 in one study and about $20,000 in the other. The third study assessed second line treatment with docetaxel, pemetrexed, and erlotinib. That analysis assumed that survival with all 3 treatments was equal, but that there was a very slight advantage in QALYs for erlotinib due to fewer adverse events. That, plus the oral administration of erlotinib, led to the finding that erlotinib second line treatment is more cost-effective than pemetrexed or docetaxel. It is unclear whether or not EGFR mutation status or cell histology was considered in this analysis.

Our search identified 7 cost-effectiveness analyses of second line treatment published since 2010. Of these, two analyses assessed erlotinib compared to docetaxel,[181, 184] two analyses assessed the gefitinib compared to docetaxel using data from the INTEREST trial,[185, 186] two analyses assessed pemetrexed versus docetaxel,[183, 187] and one analysis assessed erlotinib compared to placebo using data from the BR.21 trial.[182]

The assessment of erlotinib compared to placebo used data from the BR.21 study and the actual resource use of the patients enrolled in the trial.[182] Resources were converted into Canadian health care costs. Discounting was not used because median survival was only 1 year. The principal finding was the incremental cost-effectiveness ratio of adding erlotinib was $94,000 (Canadian) for life-year gained. In sensitivity analyses, the main driver was the magnitude of the survival benefit. Particular subgroups had more favorable ICERs, corresponding to the increased effectiveness of erlotinib in these subgroups: never smoked = $39,000; EGFR protein expression positive = $64,000; EGFR gene copy number high = $33,000. The authors concluded that "erlotinib treatment is…marginally cost-effective. The use of molecular predictors of benefit for targeted agents may help identify more or less cost-effective subgroups for treatment." The publication states that the analysis was supported by the University of Toronto.

The two analyses comparing erlotinib to docetaxel used different data sources and reached somewhat different conclusions. The first study was supported by the maker of erlotinib and used data from the BR.21 study to estimate the benefits of erlotinib and data from the TAX317 study to estimate the benefits of docetaxel, and concluded that erlotinib had a small reduction in UK National Health Services costs relative to docetaxel.[181] The second study was supported by the Canadian Center for Applied Research in Cancer Control and used observational data from patients treated in British Columbia.[184] This study found that the difference in mean overall survival between patients treated with erlotinib or docetaxel was 1 day, and the mean difference in cost was less than $3000; neither difference was statistically significant. The authors concluded that "erlotinib and docetaxel are statistically equivalent in terms of treatment cost and overall survival."

The two analyses of the comparing gefitinib to docetaxel both used data from the INTEREST trial for their estimates of effectiveness. One study was supported by two hospitals in Toronto,[185] while the other does not state how it was supported.[186] The latter study used a Thai payer perspective and concluded the gefitinib is cost-saving compared to docetaxel. The former study used the Canadian health care system perspective, and found an increase in costs with gefitinib use ($5161 per patient). The main driver of cost was the cost of the drug. No incremental cost-effectiveness ratio, in terms of life-years or QALYs, was presented. The authors concluded that "the modest increase in cost associated with gefitinib supports its use as an alternative to docetaxel as second-line treatment of advanced NSCLC."

The two analyses comparing docetaxel to pemetrexed were both supported by the makers of the drugs in question. The analysis supported by the maker of docetaxel concluded that "second line treatment for NSCLC is more cost-effective with docetaxel that with pemetrexed."[187] The analysis supported by the maker of pemetrexed concluded that "pemetrexed as a second-line treatment option for patients with a predominantly non-squamous histology in NSCLC is a cost-effective alternative to docetaxel."[183]

Key Sub-question 4.4. Which approach is more cost-effective: switch maintenance with pemetrexed, continuation maintenance therapy with pemetrexed or erlotinib?

Only one cost-effectiveness analysis was included in the review by Bongers and colleagues, published in 2010, and we also include it in our assessment here.[188] We identified 6 cost-effectiveness analyses of maintenance therapy published since 2010. Of these, 2 analyses assessed erlotinib,[189, 190] 2 assessed pemetrexed,[188, 191] and 2 assessed erlotinib compared to pemetrexed.[192, 193] All but one study were supported by the manufacturers of either erlotinib or pemetrexed. The two studies of erlotinib funded by the makers of erlotinib concluded that "erlotinib is a cost-effective treatment option when used as first-line maintenance therapy for locally advanced or metastatic NSCLC"[189] and "the overall budget impact to a health plan of expanding the use of erlotinib from the second/third line advanced NSCLC setting to include the maintenance setting was relatively small".[190] The one analysis supported by the maker of pemetrexed concluded that "compared with observation and other agents used and/or reimbursed for maintenance therapy in advanced NCSLC, pemetrexed may be considered cost-effective, particularly in patients with non-squamous cell histology."[188] The two analyses comparing erlotinib to pemetrexed, both of which were supported by the maker of erlotinib, concluded "erlotinib appears to be a cost-saving treatment alternative to pemetrexed, producing comparable survival benefits, based on indirect comparisons, at a lower cost"[193] and "erlotinib maintenance therapy in patients with advanced NSCLC causes lower adverse event management costs than pemetrexed maintenance therapy indicating a potentially superior tolerability profile".[192]

The one study that was not industry supported came from Swiss researchers and assessed the incremental cost-effectiveness ratio of adding pemetrexed to best supportive care, compared to best supportive care alone.[191] Data came from the study by Ciuleanu.[164] The model used a life-time cost horizon using a Swiss health care perspective. No discount rate was used. The principal results were that the addition of pemetrexed resulted in an incremental cost-effectiveness ratio of 106,202 Euros/QALY (approximately $145,000/QALY). The results were most sensitive to assumptions about the utility of being in the stable disease state and then the costs of best supportive care in the pemetrexed-treated patients. The authors concluded that "switch maintenance therapy with pemetrexed in patients with advanced nonsquamous-cell lung cancer after standard first-line chemotherapy is not cost-effective."[191]

Additional evidence to consider for this sub-question comes from that reported in Key Question 3 in this report, about maintenance therapy. A systematic review and meta-analysis by Zhang and colleagues[3] was unable to support clinically important differences between the switch and the continuous approach to maintenance therapy, and equally unable to support clinically important differences between switch therapy with cytotoxic agents and therapy with tyrosine kinase inhibitors. Of note, the number of original trials for assessment are small, and there are no published head-to-head comparisons of maintenance therapy with erlotinib compared to pemetrexed, meaning any conclusions must be made on indirect comparisons.

Summary of Key Question 4

There are a large number of published cost-effectiveness analyses, but approximately two-thirds of such studies are supported by the makers of the drugs being assessed. Invariably, studies supported by the makers concluded that their drug was cost-effective. Of the cost-effectiveness analyses not supported by industry, the addition of bevacizumab to first-line therapy was found in one study to be not cost-effective, erlotinib was found in one study to be marginally cost-effective, and the differences between erlotinib and docetaxel maintenance therapy were slight in another study (GRADE=low).

SUMMARY AND DISCUSSION

SUMMARY OF EVIDENCE BY KEY QUESTION

Key Question 1. First-line therapy

- **Key Sub-question 1.1.** New trials continue to support the conclusion by the CCO that any differences in survival between platinum-based doublets are modest (GRADE=High).
- **Key Sub-question 1.2.** This result continues to support the conclusions by the CCO that doublet chemotherapy including a platinum agent has a higher survival rate and a higher response rate than a single agent (GRADE=High).
- **Key Sub-question 1.3.** New trials continue to support the conclusion by Goffin and colleagues that any differences in outcomes between platinum-based agents are modest (GRADE=High).
- **Key Sub-question 1.4.** New trials continue to support the conclusion by the CCO that doublet chemotherapy including a platinum agent probably has a slight advantage over nonplatinum doublets (GRADE=moderate).
- **Key Sub-question 1.5.** One new trial does not alter the conclusion by the CCO that cisplatin combinations may have a slight advantage over carboplatin combinations in terms of survival and response rate. However, carboplatin generally has a milder toxicity than cisplatin (GRADE=moderate).
- **Key Sub-question 1.6.** New trials continue to support the review by the CCO that triplet cytotoxic therapy might have some slight advantages in terms of response rate but at an increased risk of toxicity (GRADE=High).
- **Key Sub-question 1.7.** New trials of a number of novel targeted agents have so far failed to find results equivalent to the increases in progression-free survival seen with erlotinib (mostly in patients who have never smoked) and bevacizumab (in an Asian population subgroup analysis) in the CCO review (GRADE=moderate).
- **Key Sub-question 1.7.1** Erlotinib or gefitinib monotherapy is in general superior in terms of beneficial outcomes and adverse events than cytotoxic chemotherapy in patients with EGFR mutations (GRADE=high).
- **Key Sub-question 1.12.** With the exception of studies of gefitinib and erlotinib monotherapy (in patients with EGFR mutations), doublet chemotherapy probably has a slight benefit in terms of survival compared to singlet therapy, but causes more toxicity (GRADE=moderate). Also, there now has been one trial of platinum therapy in the elderly taken to completion that found a near-doubling of the proportion of patients alive at one year in the doublet therapy group compared to monotherapy.

Summary of Key Question 2: Second-line therapy

The conclusions from the seven systematic reviews can be summarized as:

- doublet second line cytotoxic therapy might offer slight benefits in progression-free survival and response rate, not overall survival, but at a cost of increased toxicity;
- erlotinib produces modest increases in overall survival; and
- in one phase II study, the addition of bevacizumab to second line treatment resulted in improvements in survival that were not statistically significant.

The summary of these trials not included in existing systematic reviews is:

- Considering data from first line and maintenance therapy studies in addition to second line studies, there are sufficient data to support the conclusion that histology type influences the effectiveness of potential treatments. Pemetrexed is more effective in nonsquamous NSCLC, while docetaxel is more effective in squamous NSCLC (GRADE=moderate).
- Tyrosine kinase inhibitors, when used as second-line therapy in patients unselected for EGFR mutation status, produce overall survival similar to docetaxel (GRADE=strong).
- There is insufficient data to support effectiveness of other drugs, or drugs in combinations, in second-line therapy (GRADE=moderate).
- The above second line studies are typically undertaken after evidence of disease progression, and should be distinguished from mainenance therapy, which is undertaken when a patient has at least stable disease during treatment (typically four cycles).

Summary of Key Question 3: Maintenance Therapy

- Maintenance therapy improves overall survival (GRADE=high).
  - Maintenance therapy with gefitinib significantly prolonged preogression-free survival compared with placebo in patients from east Asia with advanced NSCLC who achieved disease control after first-line chemotherapy (GRADE=high).
- There is insufficient evidence to reach conclusions regarding whether a continuous or a switch strategy is superior (GRADE=very low). However, two drugs have been approved for switch therapy.
- Differences in survival in placebo-controlled trials of erlotinib or cytotoxic agents are sufficiently small that head-to-head comparisons will be required before strong conclusions can be reached about comparative effectiveness.

Summary of Key Question 4: Cost-Effectiveness Analyses

There are a large number of published cost-effectiveness analyses, but approximately two-thirds of such studies are supported by the makers of the drugs being assessed. Invariably, studies supported by the makers concluded that their drug was cost-effective. Of the cost-effectiveness analyses not supported by industry, the addition of bevacizumab to first-line therapy was found in one study to be not cost-effective, erlotinib was found in one study to be marginally cost-effective, and the differences between erlotinib and docetaxel maintenance therapy were slight in another study (GRADE=low).

LIMITATIONS

- Some comparisons of interest have not been studied in direct head-to-head studies, leaving comparisons to be made using indirect methods. Such indirect methods are highly susceptible to bias and are less reliable when differences between agents are small, as in this review.
- There is a paucity of cost-effectiveness analyses by someone other than the maker of the drug.

SUMMARY

Despite a great many new clinical trials published since 2007, evidence continues to support most of the NCCN guidelines as reported in the topic nomination brief.

Topic Nomination Brief Statement about NCCN Guidelines for First-Line Therapy of NSCLC	New Evidence
All chemotherapy regimens recommended on the NCCN website involve the use of cisplatin (or carboplatinum when cisplatinum is not tolerated).	Platinum doublets remain the standard of care. The exception would be EGFR mutation positive patients, for whom erlotinib or gefitinib monotherapy provides superior progression-free survival and fewer serious side effects.
Bevacizumab +chemotherapy or chemotherapy alone for performance status (PS) 0-1 \	The addition of bevacizumab probably yields added benefit, but with increased cost and toxicity. One cost-effectiveness analysis estimated the incremental cost-effectiveness ratio of adding bevacizumab at $560,000 per QALY gained.
Cetuximab + vinorelbine/cisplatin is also an option for PS 0-1	We identified only one new trial of cetuximab, in combination with standard chemotherapy, reporting no additional benefit.
The guidelines note that there is superior efficacy and decreased toxicity with cisplatin/pemetrexed in patients with non-squamous histology when compared with cisplatin/gemcitabine	Pemetrexed is clearly less active in squamous histology cancers. While not conclusively proven, data support the conclusion that pemetrexed is probably the preferable agent in non-squamous histology.
They also note that there is superior efficacy for cisplatin/gemcitabine in patients with squamous pathology when compared to cisplatin/pemetrexed	
Two cytotoxic agents are recommended----the guidelines state that 3 increases response rates but not survival	New systematic reviews and new trials of triplet therapy report increases in response rate and toxicity compared to doublet therapy, but has not increased overall survival.
Single agent therapy or platinum based therapy are reasonable alternatives in PS 2 patients or elderly patients	New studies suggest doublet therapy might slightly increase survival in elderly patients, but with increased toxicity.
In locally advanced NSCLC, concurrent chemotherapy and thoracic radiation (RT) is superior to RT alone and sequential chemo followed by RT	We did not look at evidence on radiation therapy.
New agent/nonplatinum combinations are reasonable alternatives if data show activity and tolerable toxicity	New evidence supports that differences between doublet therapies, whether platinum-based or otherwise, are modest.
Erlotinib is indicated as a first-line therapy in patients with EGFR mutations	This conclusion is strongly supported by new evidence.
Crizotinib is indicated as a first-line therapy in patients that are ALK positive	We did not identify new evidence about crizotinib.

RECOMMENDATIONS FOR FUTURE RESEARCH

Since VA policy makers are greatly interested about cost-effectiveness in the VA setting a proper cost-effectiveness analysis, using VA data and adjusting the population characteristics for VA patient characteristics, is needed to reach strong conclusions about cost-effectiveness of these drugs in VA setting. Such a study should be possible by combining data from this review on effectiveness with data from VA databases on the number of patients being trated, how they are being treated, the resources used, and their outcomes. Sensitivity analysis can be used to estimate the degree to which baseline assumptions would need to change in order to reach different concusions about cost-effectiveness.

REFERENCES

1. Harris, R.E., J.R. Hebert, and E.L. Wynder, *Cancer risk in male veterans utilizing the Veterans Administration medical system.* Cancer, 1989. 64(5): p. 1160-8.

2. Goffin, J., et al., *First-line systemic chemotherapy in the treatment of advanced non-small cell lung cancer: a systematic review.* Journal of Thoracic Oncology: Official Publication of the International Association for the Study of Lung Cancer, 2010. 5(2): p. 260-74.

3. Zhang, X., et al., *Maintenance therapy with continuous or switch strategy in advanced non-small cell lung cancer: a systematic review and meta-analysis.* Chest, 2011. 140(1): p. 117-26.

4. Balshem, H., et al., *GRADE guidelines: 3. Rating the quality of evidence.* J Clin Epidemiol, 2011. 64(4): p. 401-6.

5. *Chemotherapy and supportive care versus supportive care alone for advanced non-small cell lung cancer.* Cochrane Database Syst Rev, 2010(5): p. CD007309.

6. Al-Saleh, K., C. Quinton, and P.M. Ellis, *Role of pemetrexed in advanced non-small-cell lung cancer: meta-analysis of randomized controlled trials, with histology subgroup analysis.* Curr Oncol, 2012. 19(1): p. e9-e15.

7. Bosch-Barrera, J., N. Quer, and J. Brunet, *Costs and ethical issues related to first-line treatment of metastatic non-small-cell lung cancer: considerations from a public healthcare system perspective.* Clin Lung Cancer, 2011. 12(6): p. 335-40.

8. Botrel, T.E.A., et al., *Efficacy of bevacizumab (Bev) plus chemotherapy (CT) compared to CT alone in previously untreated locally advanced or metastatic non-small cell lung cancer (NSCLC): systematic review and meta-analysis.* Lung Cancer, 2011. 74(1): p. 89-97.

9. Bria, E., et al., *Outcome of advanced NSCLC patients harboring sensitizing EGFR mutations randomized to EGFR tyrosine kinase inhibitors or chemotherapy as first-line treatment: A meta-analysis.* Annals of Oncology, 2011. 22(10): p. 2277-2285.

10. Chen, P., et al., *EGFR-targeted therapies combined with chemotherapy for treating advanced non-small-cell lung cancer: a meta-analysis.* European Journal of Clinical Pharmacology, 2011. 67(3): p. 235-43.

11. Fleeman, N., et al., *Pemetrexed for the first-line treatment of locally advanced or metastatic non-small cell lung cancer.* Health Technology Assessment (Winchester, England), 2010. 14 Suppl 1: p. 47-53.

12. Gao, G., et al., *A meta-analysis of paclitaxel-based chemotherapies administered once every week compared with once every 3 weeks first-line treatment of advanced non-small-cell lung cancer.* Lung Cancer, 2012.

13. Gao, G., et al., *Epidermal growth factor receptor-tyrosine kinase inhibitor therapy is effective as first-line treatment of advanced non-small-cell lung cancer with mutated EGFR: A meta-analysis from six phase III randomized controlled trials.* International Journal of Cancer, 2012.

14. Ibrahim, E.M., *Frontline gefitinib in advanced non-small cell lung cancer: Meta-analysis of published randomized trials.* Annals of Thoracic Medicine, 2010. 5(3): p. 153-60.

15. Ibrahim, E.M., et al., *Cetuximab-based therapy is effective in chemotherapy-naive patients with advanced and metastatic non-small-cell lung cancer: a meta-analysis of randomized controlled trials.* Lung, 2011. 189(3): p. 193-8.

16. Ku, G.Y., B.A. Haaland, and G. de Lima Lopes, Jr., *Gefitinib vs. chemotherapy as first-line therapy in advanced non-small cell lung cancer: meta-analysis of phase III trials.* Lung Cancer, 2011. 74(3): p. 469-73.

17. Li, C., et al., *Gemcitabine plus paclitaxel versus carboplatin plus either gemcitabine or paclitaxel in advanced non-small-cell lung cancer: a literature-based meta-analysis.* Lung, 2010. 188(5): p. 359-64.

18. Liang, H.Y., et al., *Chemo-radiotherapy for advanced non-small cell lung cancer: concurrent or sequential? It's no longer the question: a systematic review.* Int J Cancer, 2010. 127(3): p. 718-28.

19. Lin, H., et al., *Chemotherapy with cetuximab or chemotherapy alone for untreated advanced non-small-cell lung cancer: a systematic review and meta-analysis.* Lung Cancer, 2010. 70(1): p. 57-62.

20. Mountzios, G. and K.N. Syrigos, *A benefit-risk assessment of erlotinib in non-small-cell lung cancer and pancreatic cancer.* Drug Safety, 2011. 34(3): p. 175-86.

21. Petrelli, F., et al., *Efficacy of EGFR tyrosine kinase inhibitors in patients with EGFR-mutated non-small-cell lung cancer: a meta-analysis of 13 randomized trials.* Clinical Lung Cancer, 2012. 13(2): p. 107-14.

22. Wang, F., et al., *Gefitinib Compared with Systemic Chemotherapy as First-line Treatment for Chemotherapy-naive Patients with Advanced Non-small Cell Lung Cancer: A Meta-analysis of Randomised Controlled Trials.* Clinical Oncology, 2011.

23. Yu, Y., et al., *Nonplatinum regimens of gemcitabine plus docetaxel versus platinum-based regimens in first-line treatment of advanced non-small cell lung cancer: a meta-analysis on 9 randomized controlled trials.* Cancer Chemotherapy and Pharmacology, 2012: p. 1-11.

24. Azim, H.A., Jr., et al., *Third generation triplet cytotoxic chemotherapy in advanced non-small cell lung cancer: a systematic overview.* Lung Cancer, 2009. 64(2): p. 194-8.

25. Kosmidis, P.A., et al., *Paclitaxel and gemcitabine versus paclitaxel and vinorelbine in patients with advanced non-small-cell lung cancer. A phase III study of the Hellenic Cooperative Oncology Group (HeCOG).* Annals of Oncology, 2011. 22(4): p. 827-34.

26. Shea, B.J., et al., *Development of AMSTAR: a measurement tool to assess the methodological quality of systematic reviews.* BMC Med Res Methodol, 2007. 7: p. 10.

27. Baggstrom, M.Q., et al., *Third-generation chemotherapy agents in the treatment of advanced non-small cell lung cancer: a meta-analysis.* Journal of Thoracic Oncology: Official Publication of the International Association for the Study of Lung Cancer, 2007. 2(9): p. 845-53.

28. Belani, C.P., et al., *Randomized phase III trial comparing cisplatin-etoposide to carboplatin-paclitaxel in advanced or metastatic non-small cell lung cancer.* Ann Oncol, 2005. 16(7): p. 1069-75.

29. Ichinose, Y., et al., *A multicenter randomized phase III trial of docetaxel + cisplatin (DP) vs. vindesine + cisplatin (VP) in patients with untreated stage IV non-small cell lung cancer (NSCLC) (abstract).* Ann Oncol, 2002. 13(suppl 5): p. 132-133.

30. Kim, J.H., et al., *Randomized phase II study of gemcitabine plus cisplatin versus etoposide plus cisplatin for the treatment of locally advanced or metastatic non-small cell lung cancer: Korean Cancer Study Group experience.* Lung Cancer, 2006. 52(1): p. 75-81.

31. Park, H.S., et al., *Randomized trial of docetaxel plus cisplatin (DC) versus etoposide plus cisplatin (EC) in locally advanced, recurrent, or metastatic non-small cell lung cancer (NSCLC) (abstract).* European Journal of Cancer, 2003. 1: p. S240.

32. Takiguchi, Y., et al., *The final results of a randomized phase III trial comparing irinotecan (CPT-11) and cisplatin (CDDP) with vindesine (VDS) and CDDP in advanced non-small cell lung cancer (NSCLC).* Lung Cancer, 2000. 29(Suppl 1): p. 28-29.

33. Schmittel, A., et al., *A German multicenter, randomized phase III trial comparing irinotecan-carboplatin with etoposide-carboplatin as first-line therapy for extensive-disease small-cell lung cancer.* Annals of Oncology, 2011. 22(8): p. 1798-804.

34. Zatloukal, P., et al., *A multicenter international randomized phase III study comparing cisplatin in combination with irinotecan or etoposide in previously untreated small-cell lung cancer patients with extensive disease.* Annals of Oncology, 2010. 21(9): p. 1810-6.

35. Yamamoto, N., et al., *Phase III study comparing second- and third-generation regimens with concurrent thoracic radiotherapy in patients with unresectable stage III non-small-cell lung cancer: West Japan Thoracic Oncology Group WJTOG0105.* Journal of Clinical Oncology, 2010. 28(23): p. 3739-45.

36. Socinski, M.A., et al., *Phase III study of pemetrexed plus carboplatin compared with etoposide plus carboplatin in chemotherapy-naive patients with extensive-stage small-cell lung cancer.* Journal of Clinical Oncology, 2009. 27(28): p. 4787-92.

37. Lee, S.M., et al., *Comparison of gemcitabine and carboplatin versus cisplatin and etoposide for patients with poor-prognosis small cell lung cancer.* Thorax, 2009. 64(1): p. 75-80.

38. Dimitroulis, J., et al., *Comparison of cisplatin-paclitaxel combination versus cisplatin-etoposide in patients with small-cell lung cancer: a Phase III study.* Oncology Reports, 2008. 20(4): p. 879-84.

39. Hermes, A., et al., *Irinotecan plus carboplatin versus oral etoposide plus carboplatin in extensive small-cell lung cancer: a randomized phase III trial.* Journal of Clinical Oncology, 2008. 26(26): p. 4261-7.

40. Hotta, K., et al., *Addition of platinum compounds to a new agent in patients with advanced non-small-cell lung cancer: a literature based meta-analysis of randomised trials.* Ann Oncol, 2004. 15(12): p. 1782-9.

41. Reynolds, C., et al., *Randomized phase III trial of gemcitabine-based chemotherapy with in situ RRM1 and ERCC1 protein levels for response prediction in non-small-cell lung cancer.* Journal of Clinical Oncology, 2009. 27(34): p. 5808-15.

42. Lilenbaum, R., et al., *A randomized phase III trial of single-agent pemetrexed (P) versus carboplatin and pemetrexed (CP) in patients with advanced non-small cell lung cancer (NSCLC) and performance status (PS) of 2.* J Clin Oncol, 2012. 30(suppl 2012 ASCO Annual Meeting abstracts): p. abstr 7506.

43. Le Chevalier, T., et al., *Efficacy of gemcitabine plus platinum chemotherapy compared with other platinum containing regimens in advanced non-small-cell lung cancer: a meta-analysis of survival outcomes.* Lung Cancer, 2005. 47(1): p. 69-80.

44. Douillard, J.Y., et al., *Comparison of docetaxel- and vinca alkaloid-based chemotherapy in the first-line treatment of advanced non-small cell lung cancer: a meta-analysis of seven randomized clinical trials.* J Thorac Oncol, 2007. 2(10): p. 939-46.

45. Schiller, J.H., et al., *Comparison of four chemotherapy regimens for advanced non-small-cell lung cancer.* N Engl J Med, 2002. 346(2): p. 92-8.

46. Scagliotti, G.V., et al., *Phase III randomized trial comparing three platinum-based doublets in advanced non-small-cell lung cancer.* J Clin Oncol, 2002. 20(21): p. 4285-91.

47. Rubio, J.E. and G. Shahagun, *A randomized phase III trial comparing docetaxel + carboplatin (DCP) vs vinorelbine + carboplatin (VCP) in non small cell lung cancer (NSCLC) stage III and IV (abstract).* Proc Am Soc Clin Oncol, 2003. 22: p. 703.

48. Martoni, A., et al., *Multicentre randomised phase III study comparing the same dose and schedule of cisplatin plus the same schedule of vinorelbine or gemcitabine in advanced non-small cell lung cancer.* Eur J Cancer, 2005. 41(1): p. 81-92.

49. Gebbia, V., et al., *Gemcitabine and cisplatin versus vinorelbine and cisplatin versus ifosfamide+gemcitabine followed by vinorelbine and cisplatin versus vinorelbine and cisplatin followed by ifosfamide and gemcitabine in stage IIIB-IV non small cell lung carcinoma: a prospective randomized phase III trial of the Gruppo Oncologico Italia Meridionale.* Lung Cancer, 2003. 39(2): p. 179-89.

50. Fossella, F., et al., *Randomized, multinational, phase III study of docetaxel plus platinum combinations versus vinorelbine plus cisplatin for advanced non-small-cell lung cancer: the TAX 326 study group.* J Clin Oncol, 2003. 21(16): p. 3016-24.

51. Ohe, Y., et al., *Randomized phase III study of cisplatin plus irinotecan versus carboplatin plus paclitaxel, cisplatin plus gemcitabine, and cisplatin plus vinorelbine for advanced non-small-cell lung cancer: Four-Arm Cooperative Study in Japan.* Annals of Oncology, 2007. 18(2): p. 317-23.

52. Helbekkmo, N., et al., *Vinorelbine/carboplatin vs gemcitabine/carboplatin in advanced NSCLC shows similar efficacy, but different impact of toxicity.* British Journal of Cancer, 2007. 97(3): p. 283-9.

53. Chang, J.W.-C., et al., *A randomized study of gemcitabine plus cisplatin and vinorelbine plus cisplatin in patients with advanced non-small-cell lung cancer.* Chang Gung Medical Journal, 2008. 31(6): p. 559-66.

54. Gronberg, B.H., et al., *Phase III study by the Norwegian lung cancer study group: pemetrexed plus carboplatin compared with gemcitabine plus carboplatin as first-line chemotherapy in advanced non-small-cell lung cancer.* Journal of Clinical Oncology, 2009. 27(19): p. 3217-24.

55. Okamoto, I., et al., *Phase III trial comparing oral S-1 plus carboplatin with paclitaxel plus carboplatin in chemotherapy-naive patients with advanced non-small-cell lung cancer: results of a west Japan oncology group study.* Journal of Clinical Oncology, 2010. 28(36): p. 5240-6.

56. Rodrigues-Pereira, J., et al., *A randomized phase 3 trial comparing pemetrexed/carboplatin and docetaxel/carboplatin as first-line treatment for advanced, nonsquamous non-small cell lung cancer.* Journal of Thoracic Oncology: Official Publication of the International Association for the Study of Lung Cancer, 2011. 6(11): p. 1907-14.

57. Scagliotti, G.V., et al., *Phase III study comparing cisplatin plus gemcitabine with cisplatin plus pemetrexed in chemotherapy-naive patients with advanced-stage non-small-cell lung cancer.* Journal of Clinical Oncology, 2008. 26(21): p. 3543-51.

58. Tan, E.H., et al., *Global Lung Oncology Branch trial 3 (GLOB3): final results of a randomised multinational phase III study alternating oral and i.v. vinorelbine plus cisplatin versus docetaxel plus cisplatin as first-line treatment of advanced non-small-cell lung cancer.* Annals of Oncology, 2009. 20(7): p. 1249-56.

59. Treat, J.A., et al., *A randomized, phase III multicenter trial of gemcitabine in combination with carboplatin or paclitaxel versus paclitaxel plus carboplatin in patients with advanced or metastatic non-small-cell lung cancer.* Annals of Oncology, 2010. 21(3): p. 540-7.

60. Weissman, C.H., et al., *A phase III randomized trial of gemcitabine-oxaliplatin versus carboplatin-paclitaxel as first-line therapy in patients with advanced non-small cell lung cancer.* Journal of Thoracic Oncology: Official Publication of the International Association for the Study of Lung Cancer, 2011. 6(2): p. 358-64.

61. Langer, C.J., et al., *Phase III trial comparing paclitaxel poliglumex (CT-2103, PPX) in combination with carboplatin versus standard paclitaxel and carboplatin in the treatment of PS 2 patients with chemotherapy-naive advanced non-small cell lung cancer.* Journal of Thoracic Oncology: Official Publication of the International Association for the Study of Lung Cancer, 2008. 3(6): p. 623-30.

62. Blanchard, E.M., et al., *Comparison of platinum-based chemotherapy in patients older and younger than 70 years: an analysis of Southwest Oncology Group Trials 9308 and 9509.* Journal of Thoracic Oncology: Official Publication of the International Association for the Study of Lung Cancer, 2011. 6(1): p. 115-20.

63. Treat, J., et al., *Comparison of pemetrexed plus cisplatin with other first-line doublets in advanced non-small cell lung cancer (NSCLC): A combined analysis of three phase 3 trials.* Lung Cancer, 2012. 76(2): p. 222-7.

64. Kelly, K., et al., *Randomized phase III trial of paclitaxel plus carboplatin versus vinorelbine plus cisplatin in the treatment of patients with advanced non--small-cell lung cancer: a Southwest Oncology Group trial.* J Clin Oncol, 2001. 19(13): p. 3210-8.

65. D'Addario, G., et al., *Platinum-based versus nonplatinum-based chemotherapy in advanced non-small-cell lung cancer: a meta-analysis of the published literature.* J Clin Oncol, 2005. 23(13): p. 2926-36.

66. Kawahara, M., et al., *Phase III randomized study of vinorelbine (V), gemcitabine (G) followed by docetaxel (D) (VDG) versus paclitaxel (P) and carboplatin (C) (PC) in patients (pts) with advanced non-small cell lung cancer (NSCLC) (Japan Multinational Trial Organization LC00-03) [abstract].* Proc Am Soc Clin Oncol, 2006. 24: p. 367s.

67. Pujol, J.L., F. Barlesi, and J.P. Daures, *Should chemotherapy combinations for advanced non-small cell lung cancer be platinum-based? A meta-analysis of phase III randomized trials.* Lung Cancer, 2006. 51(3): p. 335-45.

68. Rigas, J., K. Dragnev, and M. Kerry, *Survival equivalence of nonplatinum-based and latinum-based chemotherapy for advanced non-small-cell lung cancer (NSCLC): the results of a multicenter internet-based phase III randomized study (D0112) (abstract).* Lung Cancer, 2005. 49: p. S35.

69. Tan, E.H., et al., *Randomized study of vinorelbine--gemcitabine versus vinorelbine--carboplatin in patients with advanced non-small cell lung cancer.* Lung Cancer, 2005. 49(2): p. 233-40.

70. Treat, J., *A randomized phase III trial of gemcitabine (G) in combination with carboplatin (C) or paclitaxel (P) versus paclitaxel plus carboplatin in advanced (stage IIIB, IV) non-small cell lung cancer (NSCLC) (abstract).* Proc Am Soc Clin Oncol, 2003. 21: p. 624.

71. Hsu, C., et al., *Gemcitabine plus conventional-dose epirubicin versus gemcitabine plus cisplatin as first-line chemotherapy for stage IIIB/IV non-small cell lung carcinoma--a randomized phase II trial.* Lung Cancer, 2008. 62(3): p. 334-43.

72. Kosmidis, P.A., et al., *Paclitaxel and gemcitabine versus carboplatin and gemcitabine in patients with advanced non-small-cell lung cancer. A phase III study of the Hellenic Cooperative Oncology Group.* Annals of Oncology, 2008. 19(1): p. 115-22.

73. Ardizzoni, A., et al., *Cisplatin- versus carboplatin-based chemotherapy in first-line treatment of advanced non-small-cell lung cancer: an individual patient data meta-analysis.* J Natl Cancer Inst, 2007. 99: p. 847-857.

74. Hotta, K., et al., *Meta-analysis of randomized clinical trials comparing Cisplatin to Carboplatin in patients with advanced non-small-cell lung cancer.* J Clin Oncol, 2004. 22(19): p. 3852-9.

75. Jiang, J., et al., *A meta-analysis of randomized controlled trials comparing carboplatin-based to cisplatin-based chemotherapy in advanced non-small cell lung cancer.* Lung Cancer, 2007. 57(3): p. 348-58.

76. Socinski, M.A., et al., *Treatment of non-small cell lung cancer, stage IV: ACCP evidence-based clinical practice guidelines (2nd edition).* Chest, 2007. 132(3 Suppl): p. 277S-289S.

77. Alberola, V., et al., *Cisplatin plus gemcitabine versus a cisplatin-based triplet versus nonplatinum sequential doublets in advanced non-small-cell lung cancer: a Spanish Lung Cancer Group phase III randomized trial.* J Clin Oncol, 2003. 21(17): p. 3207-13.

78. Booton, R., et al., *A phase III trial of docetaxel/carboplatin versus mitomycin C/ifosfamide/cisplatin (MIC) or mitomycin C/vinblastine/cisplatin (MVP) in patients with advanced non-small-cell lung cancer: a randomised multicentre trial of the British Thoracic Oncology Group (BTOG1).* Ann Oncol, 2006. 17(7): p. 1111-9.

79. Laack, E., et al., *Randomized phase III study of gemcitabine and vinorelbine versus gemcitabine, vinorelbine, and cisplatin in the treatment of advanced non-small-cell lung cancer: from the German and Swiss Lung Cancer Study Group.* J Clin Oncol, 2004. 22(12): p. 2348-56.

80. Melo, M., et al., *Results of a randomized phase III trial comparing 4 cisplatin (P)-based regimens in the treatment of locally advanced and metastatic non-small cell lung cancer (NSCLC):mitomycin/vinblastine/cisplatin (MVP) is no longer a therapeutic option (abstract)*. Proc Am Soc Clin Oncol, 2002. 21: p. 302a.

81. Sculier, J.P., et al., *A three-arm phase III randomised trial comparing combinations of platinum derivatives, ifosfamide and/or gemcitabine in stage IV non-small-cell lung cancer*. Ann Oncol, 2002. 13(6): p. 874-82.

82. Souquet, P.J., et al., *GLOB-1: a prospective randomised clinical phase III trial comparing vinorelbine-cisplatin with vinorelbine-ifosfamide-cisplatin in metastatic non-small-cell lung cancer patients*. Ann Oncol, 2002. 13(12): p. 1853-61.

83. Boni, C., et al., *Triplets versus doublets, with or without cisplatin, in the first-line treatment of stage IIIB-IV non-small cell lung cancer (NSCLC) patients: a multicenter randomised factorial trial (FAST)*. British Journal of Cancer, 2012. 106(4): p. 658-65.

84. Comella, P., et al., *Efficacy of the combination of cisplatin with either gemcitabine and vinorelbine or gemcitabine and paclitaxel in the treatment of locally advanced or metastatic non-small-cell lung cancer: a phase III randomised trial of the Southern Italy Cooperative Oncology Group (SICOG 0101)*. Annals of Oncology, 2007. 18(2): p. 324-30.

85. Greco, F.A., et al., *Paclitaxel/Carboplatin/gemcitabine versus gemcitabine/vinorelbine in advanced non-small-cell lung cancer: a phase II/III study of the Minnie Pearl Cancer Research Network*. Clinical Lung Cancer, 2007. 8(8): p. 483-7.

86. Kubota, K., et al., *Vinorelbine plus gemcitabine followed by docetaxel versus carboplatin plus paclitaxel in patients with advanced non-small-cell lung cancer: a randomised, open-label, phase III study*. Lancet Oncology, 2008. 9(12): p. 1135-42.

87. Blumenschein, G.R., Jr., et al., *Phase III trial comparing carboplatin, paclitaxel, and bexarotene with carboplatin and paclitaxel in chemotherapy-naive patients with advanced or metastatic non-small-cell lung cancer: SPIRIT II*. Journal of Clinical Oncology, 2008. 26(11): p. 1879-85.

88. Goss, G.D., et al., *Randomized, double-blind trial of carboplatin and paclitaxel with either daily oral cediranib or placebo in advanced non-small-cell lung cancer: NCIC clinical trials group BR24 study*. Journal of Clinical Oncology, 2010. 28(1): p. 49-55.

89. Han, B., et al., *A multicenter, randomized, double-blind, placebo-controlled study to evaluate the efficacy of paclitaxel-carboplatin alone or with endostar for advanced non-small cell lung cancer*. Journal of Thoracic Oncology: Official Publication of the International Association for the Study of Lung Cancer, 2011. 6(6): p. 1104-9.

90. Hirsh, V., et al., *Randomized phase III trial of paclitaxel/carboplatin with or without PF-3512676 (Toll-like receptor 9 agonist) as first-line treatment for advanced non-small-cell lung cancer*. Journal of Clinical Oncology, 2011. 29(19): p. 2667-74.

91. Lynch, T.J., et al., *Cetuximab and first-line taxane/carboplatin chemotherapy in advanced non-small-cell lung cancer: results of the randomized multicenter phase III trial BMS099.* Journal of Clinical Oncology, 2010. 28(6): p. 911-7.

92. Manegold, C., et al., *A phase III randomized study of gemcitabine and cisplatin with or without PF-3512676 (TLR9 agonist) as first-line treatment of advanced non-small-cell lung cancer.* Annals of Oncology, 2012. 23(1): p. 72-7.

93. Mok, T.S.K., et al., *Efficacy of bevacizumab with cisplatin and gemcitabine in Asian patients with advanced or recurrent non-squamous non-small cell lung cancer who have not received prior chemotherapy: a substudy of the Avastin in Lung trial.[Erratum appears in Asia Pac J Clin Oncol. 2011 Sep;7(3):321 Note: Thitiya, Sirisinha [corrected to Sirisinha, Thitiya]].* Asia-Pacific Journal of Clinical Oncology, 2011. 7 Suppl 2: p. 4-12.

94. Ramlau, R., et al., *Randomized phase III trial comparing bexarotene (L1069-49)/cisplatin/vinorelbine with cisplatin/vinorelbine in chemotherapy-naive patients with advanced or metastatic non-small-cell lung cancer: SPIRIT I.* Journal of Clinical Oncology, 2008. 26(11): p. 1886-92.

95. Reck, M., et al., *Overall survival with cisplatin-gemcitabine and bevacizumab or placebo as first-line therapy for nonsquamous non-small-cell lung cancer: results from a randomised phase III trial (AVAiL).* Annals of Oncology, 2010. 21(9): p. 1804-9.

96. Scagliotti, G., et al., *Phase III study of carboplatin and paclitaxel alone or with sorafenib in advanced non-small-cell lung cancer.* Journal of Clinical Oncology, 2010. 28(11): p. 1835-42.

97. Gatzemeier, U., et al., *Phase III study of erlotinib in combination with cisplatin and gemcitabine in advanced non-small-cell lung cancer: the Tarceva Lung Cancer Investigation Trial.* Journal of Clinical Oncology, 2007. 25(12): p. 1545-52.

98. Giaccone, G., et al., *Gefitinib in combination with gemcitabine and cisplatin in advanced non-small-cell lung cancer: a phase III trial--INTACT 1.* J Clin Oncol, 2004. 22(5): p. 777-84.

99. Herbst, R.S., et al., *TRIBUTE: a phase III trial of erlotinib hydrochloride (OSI-774) combined with carboplatin and paclitaxel chemotherapy in advanced non-small-cell lung cancer.* J Clin Oncol, 2005. 23(25): p. 5892-9.

100. Herbst, R.S., et al., *Gefitinib in combination with paclitaxel and carboplatin in advanced non-small-cell lung cancer: a phase III trial--INTACT 2.* J Clin Oncol, 2004. 22(5): p. 785-94.

101. Sandler, A., et al., *Paclitaxel-carboplatin alone or with bevacizumab for non-small-cell lung cancer.* N Engl J Med, 2006. 355(24): p. 2542-50.

102. Reck, M., et al. (2009) *Phase III trial of cisplatin plus gemcitabine with either placebo or bevacizumab as first-line therapy for nonsquamous non-small-cell lung cancer: AVAil.* Journal of clinical oncology : official journal of the American Society of Clinical Oncology, 1227-34.

103. Paz-Ares, L., et al., *Phase III study of gemcitabine and cisplatin with or without aprinocarsen, a protein kinase C-alpha antisense oligonucleotide, in patients with advanced-stage non-small-cell lung cancer.* J Clin Oncol, 2006. 24(9): p. 1428-34.

104. Pirker, R., et al., *Cetuximab plus chemotherapy in patients with advanced non-small-cell lung cancer (FLEX): an open-label randomised phase III trial.* Lancet, 2009. 373(9674): p. 1525-31.

105. Gaafar, R.M., et al., *A double-blind, randomised, placebo-controlled phase III intergroup study of gefitinib in patients with advanced NSCLC, non-progressing after first line platinum-based chemotherapy (EORTC 08021/ILCP 01/03).* European Journal of Cancer, 2011. 47(15): p. 2331-40.

106. Takeda, K., et al., *Randomized phase III trial of platinum-doublet chemotherapy followed by gefitinib compared with continued platinum-doublet chemotherapy in Japanese patients with advanced non-small-cell lung cancer: results of a west Japan thoracic oncology group trial (WJTOG0203).* Journal of Clinical Oncology, 2010. 28(5): p. 753-60.

107. Thongprasert, S., et al., *Health-related quality-of-life in a randomized phase III first-line study of gefitinib versus carboplatin/paclitaxel in clinically selected patients from Asia with advanced NSCLC (IPASS).* Journal of Thoracic Oncology: Official Publication of the International Association for the Study of Lung Cancer, 2011. 6(11): p. 1872-80.

108. Mok, T.S., et al., *Gefitinib or carboplatin-paclitaxel in pulmonary adenocarcinoma.* New England Journal of Medicine, 2009. 361(10): p. 947-57.

109. Maemondo, M., et al., *Gefitinib or chemotherapy for non-small-cell lung cancer with mutated EGFR.* New England Journal of Medicine, 2010. 362(25): p. 2380-8.

110. Mitsudomi, T., et al., *Gefitinib versus cisplatin plus docetaxel in patients with non-small-cell lung cancer harbouring mutations of the epidermal growth factor receptor (WJTOG3405): an open label, randomised phase 3 trial.* Lancet Oncology, 2010. 11(2): p. 121-8.

111. Han, J.Y., et al., *First-SIGNAL: first-line single-agent iressa versus gemcitabine and cisplatin trial in never-smokers with adenocarcinoma of the lung.* J Clin Oncol, 2012. 30(10): p. 1122-8.

112. Zhou, C., et al., *Erlotinib versus chemotherapy as first-line treatment for patients with advanced EGFR mutation-positive non-small-cell lung cancer (OPTIMAL, CTONG-0802): a multicentre, open-label, randomised, phase 3 study.* Lancet Oncology, 2011. 12(8): p. 735-42.

113. Rosell, R., et al., *Erlotinib versus standard chemotherapy as first-line treatment for European patients with advanced EGFR mutation-positive non-small-cell lung cancer (EURTAC): a multicentre, open-label, randomised phase 3 trial.* Lancet Oncology, 2012. 13(3): p. 239-46.

114. Gridelli, C., et al., *First-Line Erlotinib Followed by Second-Line Cisplatin-Gemcitabine Chemotherapy in Advanced Non-Small-Cell Lung Cancer: The TORCH Randomized Trial.* J Clin Oncol, 2012. 30(24): p. 3002-11.

115. Quoix, E., et al., *Carboplatin and weekly paclitaxel doublet chemotherapy compared with monotherapy in elderly patients with advanced non-small-cell lung cancer: IFCT-0501 randomised, phase 3 trial.* Lancet, 2011. 378(9796): p. 1079-88.

116. Hainsworth, J.D., et al., *Weekly docetaxel versus docetaxel/gemcitabine in the treatment of elderly or poor performance status patients with advanced nonsmall cell lung cancer: a randomized phase 3 trial of the Minnie Pearl Cancer Research Network.* Cancer, 2007. 110(9): p. 2027-34.

117. Georgoulias, V., et al., *Docetaxel versus docetaxel plus gemcitabine as front-line treatment of patients with advanced non-small cell lung cancer: a randomized, multicenter phase III trial.* Lung Cancer, 2008. 59(1): p. 57-63.

118. Comella, P., et al., *Gemcitabine with either paclitaxel or vinorelbine vs paclitaxel or gemcitabine alone for elderly or unfit advanced non-small-cell lung cancer patients.* Br J Cancer, 2004. 91(3): p. 489-97.

119. Gridelli, C., et al., *Chemotherapy for elderly patients with advanced non-small-cell lung cancer: the Multicenter Italian Lung Cancer in the Elderly Study (MILES) phase III randomized trial.* J Natl Cancer Inst, 2003. 95(5): p. 362-72.

120. Kudoh, S., et al., *Phase III study of docetaxel compared with vinorelbine in elderly patients with advanced non-small-cell lung cancer: results of the West Japan Thoracic Oncology Group Trial (WJTOG 9904).* J Clin Oncol, 2006. 24(22): p. 3657-63.

121. Georgoulias, V., et al., *Vinorelbine plus cisplatin versus docetaxel plus gemcitabine in advanced non-small-cell lung cancer: a phase III randomized trial.* J Clin Oncol, 2005. 23(13): p. 2937-45.

122. Kosmidis, P., et al., *Paclitaxel plus carboplatin versus gemcitabine plus paclitaxel in advanced non-small-cell lung cancer: a phase III randomized trial.* J Clin Oncol, 2002. 20(17): p. 3578-85.

123. Shepherd, F.A., et al., *Prospective randomized trial of docetaxel versus best supportive care in patients with non-small-cell lung cancer previously treated with platinum-based chemotherapy.* J Clin Oncol, 2000. 18(10): p. 2095-103.

124. Qi, W.X., et al., *Effectiveness and safety of pemetrexed-based doublet versus pemetrexed alone as second-line treatment for advanced non-small-cell lung cancer: a systematic review and meta-analysis.* J Cancer Res Clin Oncol, 2012.

125. Qi, W.-X., et al., *The role of vandetanib in the second-line treatment for advanced non-small-cell-lung cancer: a meta-analysis of four randomized controlled trials.* Lung, 2011. 189(6): p. 437-43.

126. Qi, W.-X., Z. Shen, and Y. Yao, *Meta-analysis of docetaxel-based doublet versus docetaxel alone as second-line treatment for advanced non-small-cell lung cancer.* Cancer Chemotherapy & Pharmacology, 2012. 69(1): p. 99-106.

127. Yang, K., et al., *Effectiveness and safety of bevacizumab for unresectable non-small-cell lung cancer: a meta-analysis.* Clinical Drug Investigation, 2010. 30(4): p. 229-41.

128. Herbst, R.S., et al., *Phase II study of efficacy and safety of bevacizumab in combination with chemotherapy or erlotinib compared with chemotherapy alone for treatment of recurrent or refractory non small-cell lung cancer.* J Clin Oncol, 2007. 25(30): p. 4743-50.

129. Johnson, D.H., et al., *Randomized phase II trial comparing bevacizumab plus carboplatin and paclitaxel with carboplatin and paclitaxel alone in previously untreated locally advanced or metastatic non-small-cell lung cancer.* J Clin Oncol, 2004. 22(11): p. 2184-91.

130. Shepherd, F.A., et al., *Erlotinib in previously treated non-small-cell lung cancer.* N Engl J Med, 2005. 353(2): p. 123-32.

131. Di Maio, M., et al., *Individual patient data meta-analysis of docetaxel administered once every 3 weeks compared with once every week second-line treatment of advanced non-small-cell lung cancer.* Journal of Clinical Oncology, 2007. 25(11): p. 1377-82.

132. Di Maio, M., et al., *Meta-analysis of single-agent chemotherapy compared with combination chemotherapy as second-line treatment of advanced non-small-cell lung cancer.* J Clin Oncol, 2009. 27(11): p. 1836-43.

133. Gebbia, V., et al., *Weekly docetaxel vs. docetaxel-based combination chemotherapy as second-line treatment of advanced non-small-cell lung cancer patients. The DISTAL-2 randomized trial.* Lung Cancer, 2009. 63(2): p. 251-8.

134. Takeda, K., et al., *Phase III trial of docetaxel plus gemcitabine versus docetaxel in second-line treatment for non-small-cell lung cancer: results of a Japan Clinical Oncology Group trial (JCOG0104).* Annals of Oncology, 2009. 20(5): p. 835-41.

135. Pallis, A.G., et al., *A randomized phase III study of the docetaxel/carboplatin combination versus docetaxel single-agent as second line treatment for patients with advanced/metastatic non-small cell lung cancer.* BMC Cancer, 2010. 10: p. 633.

136. Herbst, R.S., et al., *Vandetanib plus docetaxel versus docetaxel as second-line treatment for patients with advanced non-small-cell lung cancer (ZODIAC): a double-blind, randomised, phase 3 trial.* Lancet Oncology, 2010. 11(7): p. 619-26.

137. de Boer, R.H., et al., *Vandetanib plus pemetrexed for the second-line treatment of advanced non-small-cell lung cancer: a randomized, double-blind phase III trial.* Journal of Clinical Oncology, 2011. 29(8): p. 1067-74.

138. Natale, R.B., et al., *Phase III trial of vandetanib compared with erlotinib in patients with previously treated advanced non-small-cell lung cancer.* Journal of Clinical Oncology, 2011. 29(8): p. 1059-66.

139. Ciuleanu, T., et al., *Efficacy and safety of erlotinib versus chemotherapy in second-line treatment of patients with advanced, non-small-cell lung cancer with poor prognosis (TITAN): a randomised multicentre, open-label, phase 3 study.* Lancet Oncology, 2012. 13(3): p. 300-8.

140. Maruyama, R., et al., *Phase III study, V-15-32, of gefitinib versus docetaxel in previously treated Japanese patients with non-small-cell lung cancer.* Journal of Clinical Oncology, 2008. 26(26): p. 4244-52.

141. Kim, E.S., et al., *Gefitinib versus docetaxel in previously treated non-small-cell lung cancer (INTEREST): a randomised phase III trial.* Lancet, 2008. 372(9652): p. 1809-18.

142. Sekine, I., et al., *Quality of life and disease-related symptoms in previously treated Japanese patients with non-small-cell lung cancer: results of a randomized phase III study (V-15-32) of gefitinib versus docetaxel.* Annals of Oncology, 2009. 20(9): p. 1483-8.

143. Lee, D.H., et al., *Randomized Phase III trial of gefitinib versus docetaxel in non-small cell lung cancer patients who have previously received platinum-based chemotherapy.* Clinical Cancer Research, 2010. 16(4): p. 1307-14.

144. Herbst, R.S., et al., *Efficacy of bevacizumab plus erlotinib versus erlotinib alone in advanced non-small-cell lung cancer after failure of standard first-line chemotherapy (BeTa): a double-blind, placebo-controlled, phase 3 trial.* Lancet, 2011. 377(9780): p. 1846-54.

145. Cullen, M.H., et al., *A randomized phase III trial comparing standard and high-dose pemetrexed as second-line treatment in patients with locally advanced or metastatic non-small-cell lung cancer.* Annals of Oncology, 2008. 19(5): p. 939-45.

146. Ready, N., et al., *Double-blind, placebo-controlled, randomized phase 2 study of the proapoptotic agent AT-101 plus docetaxel, in second-line non-small cell lung cancer.* Journal of Thoracic Oncology: Official Publication of the International Association for the Study of Lung Cancer, 2011. 6(4): p. 781-5.

147. Ramlau, R., et al., *Phase III study comparing oral topotecan to intravenous docetaxel in patients with pretreated advanced non-small-cell lung cancer.* J Clin Oncol, 2006. 24(18): p. 2800-7.

148. Paz-Ares, L., et al., *Phase III trial comparing paclitaxel poliglumex vs docetaxel in the second-line treatment of non-small-cell lung cancer.* British Journal of Cancer, 2008. 98(10): p. 1608-13.

149. Krzakowski, M., et al., *Phase III trial comparing vinflunine with docetaxel in second-line advanced non-small-cell lung cancer previously treated with platinum-containing chemotherapy.* Journal of Clinical Oncology, 2010. 28(13): p. 2167-73.

150. Schiller, J.H., et al., *Pemetrexed with or without matuzumab as second-line treatment for patients with stage IIIB/IV non-small cell lung cancer.* Journal of Thoracic Oncology: Official Publication of the International Association for the Study of Lung Cancer, 2010. 5(12): p. 1977-85.

151. Fossella, F.V., et al., *Randomized phase III trial of docetaxel versus vinorelbine or ifosfamide in patients with advanced non-small-cell lung cancer previously treated with platinum-containing chemotherapy regimens. The TAX 320 Non-Small Cell Lung Cancer Study Group.* J Clin Oncol, 2000. 18(12): p. 2354-62.

152. Garassino, M.C., et al., *TAILOR: A phase III trial comparing erlotinib with docetaxel as the second-line treatment of NSCLC patients with wild-type (wt) EGFR.* J Clin Oncol, 2012. 30(suppl 2012 ASCO Annual Meeting): p. abstr LBA7501.

153. Von Pawel, J., et al., *A randomized phase II study of pemetrexed versus pemetrexed plus erlotinib in second-line treatment for locally advanced or metastatic, nonsquamous NSCLC.* J Clin Oncol, 2011. 29(suppl 2011 ASCO Annual Meeting): p. abstr 7526.

154. Tan, F., et al., *Icotinib (BPI-2009H), a novel EGFR tyrosine kinase inhibitor, displays potent efficacy in preclinical studies.* Lung Cancer, 2012. 76(2): p. 177-82.

155. Cappuzzo, F., et al., *Erlotinib as maintenance treatment in advanced non-small-cell lung cancer: a multicentre, randomised, placebo-controlled phase 3 study.* Lancet Oncology, 2010. 11(6): p. 521-9.

156. Qi, W.-X., et al., *Erlotinib and pemetrexed as maintenance therapy for advanced non-small-cell lung cancer: a systematic review and indirect comparison.* Current Medical Research & Opinion, 2012. 28(4): p. 643-50.

157. Brodowicz, T., et al., *Cisplatin and gemcitabine first-line chemotherapy followed by maintenance gemcitabine or best supportive care in advanced non-small cell lung cancer: a phase III trial.* Lung Cancer, 2006. 52(2): p. 155-63.

158. Belani, C.P., et al., *Phase III study of maintenance gemcitabine (G) and best supportive care (BSC) versus BSC, following standard combination therapy with gemcitabine-carboplatin (G-Cb) for patients with advanced non-small cell lung cancer (NSCLC).* J Clin Oncol, 2010. 28(15s): p. supple; abstr 7506.

159. Perol, M., et al., *Maintenance with either gemcitabine or erlotinib versus observation with predefined second-line treatment after cisplatin-gemcitabine induction chemotherapy in advanced NSCLC: IFCT-GFPC 0502 phase III study.* J Clin Oncol, 2010. 28(15s): p. suppl; abstr 7507.

160. Brugger, W., et al., *Prospective molecular marker analyses of EGFR and KRAS from a randomized, placebo-controlled study of erlotinib maintenance therapy in advanced non-small-cell lung cancer.* Journal of Clinical Oncology, 2011. 29(31): p. 4113-20.

161. Miller, V.A., A. Das, and M. Rossi (2009) *A randomized, double-blind, placebo-controlled, phase IIIb trial (ATLAS) comparing bevacizumab (B) therapy with or without erlotinib (E) after completion of chemotherapy with B for first-line treatment of locally advanced, recurrent, or metastatic non-small cell lung cancer (NSCLC) [abstract no. LBA8002].* Journal of Clinical Oncology: ASCO annual meeting proceedings, 407.

162. Kabbinavar, F.F., et al., *Overall survival (OS) in ATLAS, a phase IIIb trial comparing bevacizumab (B) therapy with or without erlotinib (E) after completion of chemotherapy (chemo) with B for first-line treatment of locally advanced, recurrent, or metastatic non-small cell lung cancer (NSCLC).* J Clin Oncol, 2010. 28(15s): p. suppl; abstr 7526.

163. Surmont, V.F., et al., *A double-blind, randomized, placebo-controlled phase III intergroup study of gefitinib (G) in patients (pts) with advanced NSCLC, non-progressing after first-line platinum-based chemotherapy (EORTC 08021-ILCP 01/03) [abstract].* Ann Oncol, 2010. 21 (suppl 8): p. viii 124.

164. Ciuleanu, T., et al., *Maintenance pemetrexed plus best supportive care versus placebo plus best supportive care for non-small-cell lung cancer: a randomised, double-blind, phase 3 study.* Lancet, 2009. 374(9699): p. 1432-40.

165. Fidias, P.M., et al., *Phase III study of immediate compared with delayed docetaxel after front-line therapy with gemcitabine plus carboplatin in advanced non-small-cell lung cancer.* Journal of Clinical Oncology, 2009. 27(4): p. 591-8.

166. Ciuleanu, T., et al. (2009) *Impact of induction chemotherapy on the outcome of treatment with pemetrexed in patients with advanced non-small-cell lung cancer: a retrospective analysis of a phase III trial [Abstract No. 256P].* Annals of Oncology, 98.

167. Paz-Ares, L., et al., *Maintenance therapy with pemetrexed plus best supportive care versus placebo plus best supportive care after induction therapy with pemetrexed plus cisplatin for advanced non-squamous non-small-cell lung cancer (PARAMOUNT): a double-blind, phase 3, randomised controlled trial.* Lancet Oncology, 2012. 13(3): p. 247-55.

168. Belani, C.P., et al., *Quality of life in patients with advanced non-small-cell lung cancer given maintenance treatment with pemetrexed versus placebo (H3E-MC-JMEN): results from a randomised, double-blind, phase 3 study.* Lancet Oncology, 2012. 13(3): p. 292-9.

169. Lee, S.M., et al., *Randomized double-blind placebo-controlled trial of thalidomide in combination with gemcitabine and Carboplatin in advanced non-small-cell lung cancer.* Journal of Clinical Oncology, 2009. 27(31): p. 5248-54.

170. Zhang, L., et al., *Gefitinib versus placebo as maintenance therapy in patients with locally advanced or metastatic non-small-cell lung cancer (INFORM; C-TONG 0804): a multicentre, double-blind randomised phase 3 trial.* The Lancet Oncology, 2012.

171. Paz-Ares, L., et al., *PARAMOUNT: Final overall survival (OS) results of the phase III study of maintenance pemetrexed (pem) plus best supportive care (BSC) versus placebo (plb) plus BSC immediately following induction treatment with pem plus cisplatin (cis) for advanced nonsquamous (NS) non-small cell lung cancer (NSCLC).* J Clin Oncol, 2012. 30(suppl 2012 ASCO Annual Meeting): p. abstr LBA7507.

172. Bongers, M.L., et al., *Cost effectiveness of treatment with new agents in advanced non-small-cell lung cancer: a systematic review.* Pharmacoeconomics, 2012. 30(1): p. 17-34.

173. Wu, B., et al., *Cost-effectiveness of adding rh-endostatin to first-line chemotherapy in patients with advanced non-small-cell lung cancer in China.* Clin Ther, 2011. 33(10): p. 1446-55.

174. Joerger, M., et al., *Addition of cetuximab to first-line chemotherapy in patients with advanced non-small-cell lung cancer: a cost-utility analysis.* Ann Oncol, 2011. 22(3): p. 567-74.

175. Thongprasert, S., et al., *Cost-effectiveness analysis of cisplatin plus etoposide and carboplatin plus paclitaxel in a phase III randomized trial for non-small cell lung cancer.* Asia Pac J Clin Oncol, 2011. 7(4): p. 369-75.

176. Ahn, M.J., et al., *Cost-effectiveness of bevacizumab-based therapy versus cisplatin plus pemetrexed for the first-line treatment of advanced non-squamous NSCLC in Korea and Taiwan.* Asia Pac J Clin Oncol, 2011. 7 Suppl 2: p. 22-33.

177. Stanisic, S., et al., *Societal cost savings through bevacizumab-based treatment in non-small cell lung cancer (NSCLC).* Lung Cancer, 2010. 69 Suppl 1: p. S24-30.

178. Giuliani, G., et al., *Cost-effectiveness analysis of bevacizumab versus pemetrexed for advanced non-squamous NSCLC in Italy.* Lung Cancer, 2010. 69 Suppl 1: p. S11-7.

179. Bischoff, H.G., et al., *Costs of bevacizumab and pemetrexed for advanced non-squamous NSCLC in Italy and Germany.* Lung Cancer, 2010. 69 Suppl 1: p. S18-23.

180. Goulart, B. and S. Ramsey, *A trial-based assessment of the cost-utility of bevacizumab and chemotherapy versus chemotherapy alone for advanced non-small cell lung cancer.* Value Health, 2011. 14(6): p. 836-45.

181. Lewis, G., et al., *Cost-effectiveness of erlotinib versus docetaxel for second-line treatment of advanced non-small-cell lung cancer in the United Kingdom.* J Int Med Res, 2010. 38(1): p. 9-21.

182. Bradbury, P.A., et al., *Economic analysis: randomized placebo-controlled clinical trial of erlotinib in advanced non-small cell lung cancer.* Journal of the National Cancer Institute, 2010. 102(5): p. 298-306.

183. Asukai, Y., et al., *Cost-effectiveness analysis of pemetrexed versus docetaxel in the second-line treatment of non-small cell lung cancer in Spain: results for the non-squamous histology population.* BMC Cancer. 10: p. 26.

184. Cromwell, I., et al., *Erlotinib or docetaxel for second-line treatment of non-small cell lung cancer: a real-world cost-effectiveness analysis.* J Thorac Oncol, 2011. 6(12): p. 2097-103.

185. Horgan, A.M., et al., *An economic analysis of the INTEREST trial, a randomized trial of docetaxel versus gefitinib as second-/third-line therapy in advanced non-small-cell lung cancer.* Ann Oncol, 2011. 22(8): p. 1805-11.

186. Thongprasert, S., S. Tinmanee, and U. Permsuwan, *Cost-utility and budget impact analyses of gefitinib in second-line treatment for advanced non-small cell lung cancer from Thai payer perspective.* Asia Pac J Clin Oncol, 2012. 8(1): p. 53-61.

187. Vergnenegre, A., et al., *Cost-effectiveness of second-line chemotherapy for non-small cell lung cancer: an economic, randomized, prospective, multicenter phase III trial comparing docetaxel and pemetrexed: the GFPC 05-06 study.* J Thorac Oncol, 2011. 6(1): p. 161-8.

188. Klein, R., et al., *Cost-effectiveness of pemetrexed as first-line maintenance therapy for advanced nonsquamous non-small cell lung cancer.* J Thorac Oncol, 2010. 5(8): p. 1263-72.

189. Vergnenegre, A., et al., *Cross-market cost-effectiveness analysis of erlotinib as first-line maintenance treatment for patients with stable non-small cell lung cancer.* Clinicoecon Outcomes Res, 2012. 4: p. 31-7.

190. Carlson, J.J., et al., *Budget impact of erlotinib for maintenance therapy in advanced non-small cell lung cancer.* J Med Econ, 2011. 14(2): p. 159-66.

191. Matter-Walstra, K., et al., *Cost-effectiveness of maintenance pemetrexed in patients with advanced nonsquamous-cell lung cancer from the perspective of the Swiss health care system.* Value Health, 2012. 15(1): p. 65-71.

192. Banz, K., et al., *Comparison of treatment costs of grade 3/4 adverse events associated with erlotinib or pemetrexed maintenance therapy for patients with advanced non-small-cell lung cancer (NSCLC) in Germany, France, Italy, and Spain.* Lung Cancer, 2011. 74(3): p. 529-34.

193. Nuijten, M.J., et al., *A cross-market cost comparison of erlotinib versus pemetrexed for first-line maintenance treatment of patients with locally advanced or metastatic non-small-cell lung cancer.* Lung Cancer, 2011.

APPENDIX A. SEARCH STRATEGY FOR SYSTEMATIC REVIEWS AND COST-EFFECTIVENESS ANALYSES (SEARCH #1)

TREATMENT OF METASTATIC NON-SMALL-CELL LUNG CANCER
SEARCH METHODOLOGY

SEARCH STRATEGY #1 (SYSTEMATIC REVIEWS):
DATABASE SEARCHED & TIME PERIOD COVERED:
PubMed – 1966-3/16/2012
Cochrane Database of Systematic Reviews – All years

SEARCH STRATEGY (PUBMED):
lung neoplasms OR lung cancer
AND
non-small-cell OR non-small cell OR "non small cell"
AND
metastatic* OR metastasi* OR advanced
AND
Systematic[sb]

NUMBER OF RESULTS: 436

SEARCH STRATEGY (COCHRANE):
(Lung neoplasm* OR lung cancer):ti,ab,kw
AND
(Non-small cell OR "non small cell" OR non-small-cell):ti,ab,kw

NUMBER OF RESULTS: 13

===
SEARCH STRATEGY #2 (COST-EFFECTIVENESS):
DATABASE SEARCHED & TIME PERIOD COVERED:
PubMed – 1966-3/16/2012
Cochrane Economic Evaluations – All years

PUBMED:
lung neoplasms OR lung cancer
AND
non-small-cell OR non-small cell OR "non small cell"
AND
metastatic* OR metastasi* OR advanced
AND

cost OR costs OR cost-effective* OR cost-benefit OR cost utility OR cost-utilities OR cost analysis OR cost analyses OR economic OR economics
NOT
Results of Search #1

NUMBER OF RESULTS: 347

COCHRANE
(Lung neoplasm* OR lung cancer):ti,ab,kw
AND
(Non-small cell OR "non small cell" OR non-small-cell):ti,ab,kw

NUMBER OF RESULTS: 30

APPENDIX B. SEARCH STRATEGY FOR TRIALS (SEARCH #2)

NON-SMALL CELL LUNG CANCER – RCTS SEARCH METHODOLOGY

DATABASE SEARCHED & TIME PERIOD COVERED:
Medline on OVID – 2007-5/8/2012

LANGUAGE:
English

SEARCH STRATEGY:
(systematic review? or systematic overview?).tw. OR meta-analysis/ OR meta analysis.pt. OR metaanalys$.tw. OR meta analys$.tw. OR meta-analys$.tw. OR randomized controlled trials/ or randomized controlled trial.pt. OR random allocation/OR (random$ and (trial* or stud$)).ti,ab
AND
carcinoma, non-small-cell lung/ or nscls.ti,ab.OR (lung and (cancer$ or neoplasm$ or carcinom$ or malignan$ or tumo?r$)).ti,ab.
AND
(paclitaxel or taxol or docetaxel or taxotere or gemcitabine or gemzar or vinorelbine or navelbine or irinotecan or campto or camptosar or CPT-11 or pemetrexed or alimta or erlotinib or tarceva or gefitinib or iressa or bevacizumab or avastin or cetuximab or crizotinib).ti,ab.

NUMBER OF RESULTS: 772

===

DATABASE SEARCHED & TIME PERIOD COVERED:
Embase – 2007-5/8/2012

LANGUAGE:
English

SEARCH STRATEGY:
paclitaxel:ti OR taxol:ti OR docetaxel:ti OR taxotere:ti OR gemcitabine:ti OR gemzar:ti OR vinorelbine:ti OR navelbine:ti OR irinotecan:ti OR campto:ti OR camptosar:ti OR 'cpt 11':ti OR pemetrexed:ti OR alimta:ti OR erlotinib:ti OR tarceva:ti OR gefitinib:ti OR iressa:ti OR bevacizumab:ti OR avastin:ti OR cetuximab:ti OR crizotinib:ti OR paclitaxel:ab OR taxol:ab OR docetaxel:ab OR taxotere:ab OR gemcitabine:ab OR gemzar:ab OR vinorelbine:ab OR navelbine:ab OR irinotecan:ab OR campto:ab OR camptosar:ab OR 'cpt 11':ab OR pemetrexed:ab OR alimta:ab OR erlotinib:ab OR tarceva:ab OR gefitinib:ab OR iressa:ab OR bevacizumab:ab OR avastin:ab OR cetuximab:ab OR crizotinib:ab OR 'paclitaxel'/exp OR paclitaxel
AND

((('lung'/exp AND (cancer* OR neoplasm* OR carcinoma* OR malignan* OR tumor* OR tumour*) AND non:ti OR non:ab)) OR 'lung non small cell cancer'/exp OR nsclc:ti OR nsclc:ab
AND
(randomized AND controlled AND trial*) OR (random AND allocation) OR (random* AND (trial* OR stud*))
AND
HUMAN
AND
'article'/it OR 'article in press'/it

NUMBER OF RESULTS: 659

===

DATABASE SEARCHED & TIME PERIOD COVERED:
Cochrane Register of Controlled Trials: 2007-5/8/2012

SEARCH STRATEGY:
"paclitaxel or taxol or docetaxel or taxotere or gemcitabine or gemzar or vinorelbine or navelbine or irinotecan or campto or camptosar or CPT-11 or pemetrexed or alimta or erlotinib or tarceva or gefitinib or iressa or bevacizumab or avastin or cetuximab or crizotinib in Title, Abstract or Keywords
AND
non-small cell lung OR nonsmall cell lung OR nsclc in Title, Abstract or Keywords

NUMBER OF RESULTS: 516

===

TOTAL NUMBER OF RESULTS AFTER REMOVAL OF DUPLICATES & NON-RELEVANT MATERIAL (INCLUDING PHASE II TRIALS); 820

APPENDIX C. SCREENER FORMS USED FOR SYSTEMATIC REVIEWS AND COST-EFFECTIVENESS ANALYSES

ID:
Author:

1. Is it a cost-effectiveness analysis?
    Yes .... ☐
    No .... ☐STOP

KEEP FOR BACKGROUND ☐

2. Does it present data on metastatic non-small cell lung cancer?
    Yes .... ☐
    No .... ☐STOP
    Stage I .... ☐STOP
    Stage II .... ☐STOP
    Stage III .... ☐
    Stage IV .... ☐
    "Advanced" .... ☐

NOTES

3. Which kind of therapy is assessed? (Check all that apply)
    First line .... ☐
    Second line .... ☐
    Maintenance .... ☐
    Not Stated .... ☐

4. Which treatments is assessed?
    _____

5. Where are the data from?
    Multiple studies .... ☐
    Single study .... ☐
        Name: _____

6. What perspective is the analysis?
    US payer .... ☐
    Non-US payer .... ☐
    Societal .... ☐
    _____ .... ☐

7. What outcome is used?
    QALYs .... ☐
    Life expectancy .... ☐
    _____ .... ☐

8. Conclusions per abstract:

ID:
Author:

1. Is it a systematic review?
   Yes.. ☐
   No ....☐STOP

2. Does it present data on metastatic non-small cell lung cancer?
   Yes.. ☐
   No ....☐STOP
   Stage I ....☐STOP
   Stage II ....☐STOP
   Stage III .... ☐
   Stage IV .... ☐
   "Advanced" .... ☐

3. Which kind of therapy is assessed? (Check all that apply)
   First line.................................. ☐
   Second line .... ☐
   Maintenance .... ☐
   Not Stated .... ☐

4. Which treatments are captured? None below: ☐STOP

KEEP FOR BACKGROUND ☐

6. Which databases were searched?
   Pubmed/Medline ☐   Embase ☐
   Cochrane ☐   Other ☐

7. How many studies were included?
   _____

8. What outcomes were reported?
   Overall survival .... ☐
   Progression free survival .... ☐
   Overall response rate .... ☐
   Adverse events............................... ☐
   _____
   _____
   _____

9. Conclusions per abstract:
   _____
   _____
   _____
   _____
   _____
   _____
   _____

	Bevacizumab	Cetuximab	Platinum agent/therapy	Gemcitabine+taxol	Gemcitabine+platinum	Pemetrexed	Erlotinib	Crizotinib	Endostar	Docetaxel	Ciefitinib	Vandetanib	Placebo	Immunotherapy	Paclitaxel	Gifitinib	Various
Bevacizumab																	
Cetuximab																	
Platinum agent/therapy																	
Gemcitabine+taxol																	
Gemcitabine+platinum																	
Pemetrexed																	
Erlotinib																	
Crizotinib																	
Endostar																	
Docetaxel																	
Ciefitinib																	
Vandetanib																	
Placebo																	
Immunotherapy																	
Paclitaxel																	
Gifitinib																	

NOTES:

5. What was the end date of the search?
   January .... ☐
   February .... ☐
   March .... ☐
   April .... ☐
   May .... ☐
   June .... ☐
   July .... ☐
   August .... ☐
   September .... ☐
   October .... ☐
   November .... ☐
   December................ ☐
   NS .... ☐
   2008 .... ☐
   2009 .... ☐
   2010 .... ☐
   2011 .... ☐
   NS .... ☐

APPENDIX D. PEER REVIEWER COMMENTS AND RESPONSES

Comment	Response
Pre-Results	
I note that the attribution to the 1st line guideline is Goffin et al. Similar to this VA project, I led what was a group effort. At some (or all) points, it would be appropriate to indicate that the guideline was the work of the Cancer Care Ontario Program in Evidence-Based Care (CCO PEBC or CCO)	We have updated the report to include the CCO
In the search methods, there is no indication of searching conference abstracts? Was this done.	We did not search conference abstracts
P.10 "(the exception being the same of the never…orally)": This wording in the parentheses makes no sense. What does "the exception being the same of" mean? I think you mean 'newer" targeted therapies, not 'never'	This typo has been corrected.
Key Question #1	
There is very little mention of the importance of molecular markers in the management of advanced NSCLC	Molecular markers are mentioned in the targeted therapy section. We did not identify studies using molecular markers to guide therapy outside of this area. We did identify studies that used molecular markers as a means for assessing overall prognosis, but that was not one of our key questions.
p.16 "The five additional trials…docetaxel plus cisplatin." : This is incorrect according to your table and the reference. Docetaxel plus cisplatin had superior survival over vindesine plus cisplatin.	This typo has been corrected.
Page 17. Summary 1.1. Given that survival is arguably the most important endpoint, QoL perhaps second, and others of lesser importance, I recommend specifying the "outcome" being considered as much as possible. Here it is survival.	We have specified that this is survival.
Page 18. Summary 1.2 As per 1.1, does one trial indicating a trend toward improvement with doublet negate the meta-analysis indicating survival improvement. Thus, the recommendations might continue to support a 'survival' improvement rather than just a response improvement.	We have added survival to this conclusion.
Page 18- first paragraph- New study presented at ASCO2012 by Lilenbaum, et al showed that 2 agents were better than 1 in PS 2 patients. This study has not been included in the discussion.	This study has now been included
P. 19 "There was no difference… grade 3/4 toxicities": Should be 8.6 months, not 86	This typo has been corrected.
Last paragraph of page 22- It is important to point out that in the meta-analyses by Ardizonni, et al the benefit with cisplatin compared to carboplatin was more pronounced in non-squamous patients and when combined with newer agents.	We added the data about non squamous histology.

Comment	Response
Page 24. Summary 1.5. Is it worth mentioning the differences in toxicity profiles between cisplatin and carboplatin in this palliative setting?	We have added this.
P27. Additional relevant papers for 1.7.1: Mitsudomi et al Lancet Oncol. 2010 Feb;11(2):121-8.	This study has now been included
P27. Additional relevant papers for 1.7.1: Han, JCO, 2012, 30(10):2233-28	This study has now been included
P27. Additional relevant papers for 1.7.1: Rosell et al, EURTAC, Lancet Onc 13:239-46, 2012 ß this last trial is relevant in extending the several Asian studies to a Caucasian population.	This study has now been included
Table F5 needs to be updated. There are now more studies.	This has been updated
Page 27, Summary 1.7. is confusing, as it seems to suggest an OS advantage to EGFR TKI, where this has not technically been shown. I would be clear the 'outcome' is PFS. Also, bevacizumab may or may not improvement survival in the general population. Is it specific to carboplatin and paclitaxel, and is it better in the Asian population?	We have clarified the outcome as progression-free survival and the qualifier about the Asian subgroup.
P. 27: Add ";" to "other outcomes progression-free survival of 10.1.."	This typo has been corrected.
It may also be worth specifying that in the absence of a mutation, first line tki is associated with a worse survival and should be avoided, as seen in the TORCH study. See URL: http://jco.ascopubs.org/content/early/2012/07/09/JCO.2011.41.2056.full.pdf#page=1&view=FitH	This study has now been included
Page 29, New Lit. I would rewrite this for clarity as it jumps around a bit. Opening para could indicate "2 studies found assessing cytotoxics specifically in the elderly, and 2 studies examining first line egfr tki's assessed subsets of elderly." Second para could discuss the cytotoxic studies, third the TKI's.	We have re-arranged this section.
Unsure why reference 113 Georgoulias is included in this elderly section. Median age 63 is a 'young' lung cancer population, and no subset is specified. Would remove.	We left this article in at the request of another technical expert, but added the additional qualifier about the age.
Page 30. Summary 1.12. I dispute the "Grade=low" for survival benefit. The benefit may be very modest (which is common to most NSCLC trials) but data quality is not. Looking at the 70-80 population, I highly doubt we will see a new trial indicating that a doublet is bad. Caveats about the 80+ population might be reasonable.	We agree our initial GRADE was too conservative and have reclassified to moderate based on RCT data that are sparse (only 6 trials and all of different regimens, 4 of which found a benefit for doublet therapy and 2 of which did not).
P.30 1.12 summary: You should mention here that the data for monotherapy is from subgroup analyses	This caveat has been added.
On page 30 summary of key sub-question 1.12- Please mention that the only study evaluating a platinum based combination showed a survival advantage in elderly patients compared to single agent therapy.	This addition has been made.

Comment	Response
Key Question #2	
Page 32. First sentence of the page repeats itself between its first and second clause.	This typo has been corrected.
Page 32. Existing Systemic Reviews. Re Qi review 2012: The approval or non-approval of a drug seems irrelevant to the notion efficacy. More important might be the heterogeneity of the drugs in question and the phase II nature of some of the references.	To be relevant to VA, a drug has to be FDA approved for use in the US, although not necessarily approved for the particular use in question. We revised and increased the discussion of bortezomib and vandetanib.
P.32: Only bortezomib and vandetanib are FDA approved, but not for NSCLC; the other two agents are not approved	This has been corrected.
P.32, Table on p. 34: This is misspelled here and in the Table on Page 34=bortezomib not bortezonib;	This typo has been corrected.
P. 32, p. 37, p. 38: Vandetanib is FDA approved, but not for NSCLC (also see the same statement on pages 37 and 38)	This has been corrected.
On page 32 the authors have missed the study by von Pawel, et al presented at ASCO 2011. Also please include the meta-analyses by Di Maio M, J Clin Oncol 2007.	This study has now been included
Page 32, 33 please include the TAILOR study presented at ASCO 2012 by Garassino, et al, comparing docetaxel and erlotinib	This study has now been included
Page 33. Para "The fifth system review…" appears to be a combination of first and second line studies. Also, the 'overall' survival was for which comparison? It would be useful to specify.	This has been clarified; the overall survival result comes from the BR.21 study.
Para "The conclusions…" Third bullet. Might be pointed out this was a phase II study only.	This has been added.
Page 37. Does it add value to singly review the studies which were already included in the systemic reviews already mentioned (assuming those reviews were of sufficient quality). Or does this just add document length?	We agree and have deleted the text about trials contained in existing systematic reviews that we discuss in detail in the prior section. However, we retained the description of trials that were otherwise only included in the reviews by Qi and colleagues as we did not discuss these reviews in detail.
Page 38. Para "The last of the trials…" The paragraph suggests "no significant difference" between vandetanib and erlotinib. It should then specify whether a test for non-inferiority was achieved. Otherwise they sound truly equivalent.	This was a superiority trial, which failed. Then a test for non-inferiority was done with non-inferiority defined as "at least 50% of the efficacy" of erlotinib. We have added this to the description.
Page 39. "New Agents". For these studies, it is likely useful to specify whether these were 'all comers' or 'mutation only' patients as the distinction has become relevant. Readers should know there is utility for the mutation negative population, as not all will be aware.	This has been added.

Comment	Response
Page 40 Para "Sekine and colleagues…." I would addend this to the preceding paragraph as the QoL component as it seems like a completely different study until the last sentence and adds undue length.	This change has been made.
Page 40. "Kim and colleagues…." Specifying non-inferiority vs. failed superiority will aid the audience in understanding how to use these drugs. If it is a failed superiority study only, it should not become part of the armamentarium. Similarly for other studies in this section.	We have now indicated that the primary analysis in this study was a superiority analysis, which was not statistically significant.
Page 40. Last sentence just before "Pemetrexed" section. Much higher? 13 vs. 6%.	This has been revised.
THOUGHT: for Table S2, alter the columns such that there is only one column indicating the Systemic Review Y/N: this can either be "Di Maio" "Qi 2012" etc, or "No". The other columns are freed for other items, possibly: "n" "non-inferiority comparison Y/N or p= ", "HR for OS", etc. More data, less wasted space.	This table has been revised to include only the studies in existing systematic reviews. Some of the other suggested columns are already included in Table S3, to which we have added histology and EGFR mutation status.
Page 45. Having a summary of the "trials not in reviews" in isolation is not helpful. The whole section appears to read as an unordered catalogue. A net synthesis seems is required. In fact, at the end of the second line section, a reader new to the topic will have little idea has to how they should practice. One might consider ordering it as the data built up historically: 1) it was found that docetaxel was better than best supportive care; 2) Pemetrexed was compared to docetaxel and found to be essentially equivalent but more friendly and thus caught on; 3) The EGFR TKI's were new and are even more friendly, and were thus studied. Importantly, they were studied as 2nd/3rd line vs. BSC, and thus may be kept in reserve after another second-line therapy. In any case, there is data they are equivalent to docetaxel in second line, and thus serve as an option; and 4) LUMP: other studies have been done, which have not added much to the second line notion: more ain't better; other sexy drugs haven't yet added much. Then one could give corresponding recommendations. This section could also be arranged by approved agents, citing the trials supporting the use of each, comparisons, etc, then going on to the 'other' agents.	We have reorganized this section following this suggestion.
NOTE that treatment by histology has had no mention here (it only seems to come up under cost-effectiveness). Histology now plays an important role in chemotherapy choice, particularly in 2nd/maintenance lines. The survival differences between docetaxel and pemetrexed by histology are at least as large/important as comparisons such as doublets vs. single agents. Although a portion of this data is from subsets, a document aiming to encompass 1st line, 2nd line, and maintenance is obligated to cover histology.	We have added a conclusion about pemetrexed and histology.

Comment	Response
Similar reference to histology for first line seems appropriate.	The issue of histology and pemetrexed use in first-line therapy is presented in the discussion of the prior reviews by Goffin and colleagues.
P. 47 "The erlotinib group had an overall survival… 1.09)": This should be HR=0.9, not 0.90 months; also you should include a p value of 0.2686	This has been corrected.
Key Question #3	
Table M1. 1st box under 'what was compared' gefitinib is spelled incorrectly with all i's.	This typo has been corrected.
Page 48. Just before reference 158. Cisplati is missing an 'n'.	This typo has been corrected.
P.50: I question how you rated maintenance therapy improving OS as High based on the data. For the continuous therapy there was only a trend towards benefit in OS. For the switch trials, the upper bound of the HR in all but one of the trials crossed 1	The GRADE of strong is based on the meta-analytic pooling of the trials in the Zhang meta-analysis. While each individual trial may have not yielded a statistically significant favorable result, combining them statistically did yield a statistically significant benefit for the switch strategy (HR=0.85, 95% CI: 0.79-0.92) and for continuous therapy the pooled result was a similar hazard ratio of 0.88, with a 95% CI that just crossed the null value (0.74-1.04). With the interaction being completely nonsignificant (p=0.78), the most likely explanation for the difference in the upper bound crossing the null value is fewer studies contributing to the continuous pooled analysis (n=3) than the switch pooled analysis (n=6).
P. 50 Switch therapy finding: However, there is only a trend of benefit in continuous therapy but there are two drugs approved for use for switch therapy. I think this needs to be better addressed in this entire section.	We have made this point.
Key Question #4	
Page 56. Would change "unclear whether or not EGFR receptor status" to "…not EGFR mutation status" at end of first paragraph.	This change was made.
Page 56. 2nd paragraph. The notations "(ref 498, 449)" are probably leftovers.	This typo has been corrected.
Page 59. Key sub-question 1.12. missing an 'r' in elotinib.	This typo has been corrected.
Page 61. Table comparison with NCCN. Although commonly referenced, I don't believe the NCCN 'guidelines' meet criteria for guideline quality and are more akin to consensus documents. Would a comparison with the ASCO guidelines be better?	Perhaps this would be better, but our key questions specifically mentioned the "NCCN guidelines" and that is why these are included here and referred to as "guidelines."

Comment	Response
General	
I find the answers or summaries of the Key Questions to be rather broad and lacking specific direction, making implementation difficult or impossible, therefore they are no better than the NCCN guidelines. While I appreciate the need for numerous subquestions for Key Question 1, it would be helpful for implementation to summarize the overall subquestion findings for Key Question 1 : doublets better than single, cisplatin over carbo if tolerated, pemetrexed for non-squamous histology, erlotinib for EGFR mutation, etc. I feel the summary of the maintenance therapy question needs major overhauling to make sense of the data and provide direction based on the available data.	With the exception of the "pemetrexed for nonsquamous histology," these conclusions are all currently in the report. In second-line therapy we have a conclusion that pemetrexed is more effective in nonsquamous histology. With respect to the maintenance therapy conclusions, these were formulated from the data. The peer reviewer seems to be asking for recommendations similar to those one might find in a guideline, which is not within the scope of this review.
There is very little mention of the importance of molecular markers in the management of advanced NSCLC	This has been added.
The results of the PARAMOUNT study were updated at ASCO2012. These updated results are relevant in many portions of this report.	This has been added.